Pregnancy From Conception to Birth

The Essential Roadmap for First-Time Mothers

Elizabeth Benson

information contained within this document, including, but not limited to, errors, omissions, or inaccuracies.

Table of Contents

Your children are not your children.

They are sons and daughters of Life's longing for itself.

They come through you but not from you.

And though they are with you yet they belong not to you.

You may give them your love but not your thoughts,

For they have their own thoughts.

You may house their bodies but not their souls,

For their souls dwell in the house of tomorrow, which you cannot visit, not even in your dreams.

–Kahlil Gibran

Introduction

Motherhood is a journey that begins with love and curiosity, and transforms into a never-ending story of learning, growth, and pure joy.

Pregnancy is a lot of things, but I think the overarching theme throughout those nine months is anticipation. It's like being in a constant state of wonder. From the day you find out you're pregnant, you'll be wondering what your baby will look like. As you progress, you'll be anticipating what's to come in the next month. When you eat, you might be subconsciously asking yourself if you've made a good meal choice. When you work out, you may ask yourself whether you're doing so at a safe enough pace for your baby. You're always going to want to know something.

If I were to ask you what you think the most important thing to have for a safe and happy pregnancy is, what would you say?

Would you say a healthy diet? A positive mindset?

The answer is: information. When you're clued up or reading up on pregnancy, you get to know what's happening in your body, what's normal and what's not, and how well your baby should be developing. You also get to know all the things you can do to ensure a healthy baby with ten fingers and toes.

But most importantly, you'll be able to recognize potential risks and have the confidence and knowledge to ask questions and seek prompt intervention if needed.

If you've got a litany of anxious questions, here are all the reassuring answers you need. As well as all the physical and emotional symptoms you might experience.

Most of the things that are happening to you are completely normal, but it's still nice to feel reassured and like you're on the right track.

The *journey* into parenthood has already begun. This book is a roadmap to tell you where you are, how long it takes to reach the finish line, and what happens in between. You're already a great mom.

I'm going to walk you through your pregnancy, from the time you find out, until a month and a half after your special bundle has arrived.

You'll learn more about:

- What's going on in your body?

- How your baby is developing month by month.

- The effects of certain foods and drinks on your baby and how to keep healthy throughout the pregnancy.

- The benefits of exercise, the kinds that are harmful, and the ones you should incorporate into your routine.

- How to comfortably change your lifestyle for the duration of pregnancy to ensure a healthy, bouncing baby.

- What could potentially go wrong, signs to look out for, and the recommended course of action.

- Statistics on ailments, the percentage of women they affect, and how you can either prevent or prepare for such things.

- Ways to maintain your relationships through this period and once the baby's born.

As a bonus, you'll feel like you have one more person celebrating with you.

I'm a mother myself. I've got grandchildren too, and I remember what I felt during my first pregnancy. I cherished it. I wanted to know what was going on every step of the way, and there was only one comprehensive book around at the time. I read that thing until it fell apart.

I also recall my own daughters and daughter-in-law experiencing pregnancies and exchanging some very conflicting information. It's what inspired me to seek out accurate information and put it all in one book.

Any pregnancy is beautiful, but a first pregnancy is especially wonderful. I wish I could experience it again. What you learn in this book will help to eliminate some of the anxieties that will inevitably accompany your journey into new territory. I hope it will help make a wonderful experience even better.

TRIMESTER 1:

New Adventures

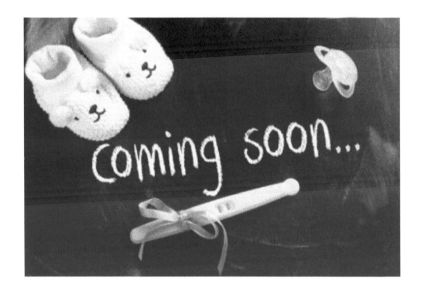

Chapter 1: Month One

You're Pregnant!

A very big congratulations to you! Here's wishing you every bit of joy that comes with being a parent—and then some!

If this news comes as a surprise and you're feeling a little unprepared, don't worry. You've got about eight more months to figure some things out. I say some because there are moms with kids in college who are still figuring things out!

There's a lot that goes on in a really short space of time when you're pregnant. As time goes on, it becomes apparent that you're sharing your body. This means you'll have to start making some changes in order to accommodate your new guest and...

It's Never Too Late to Change Your Habits

As far as changing habits go, I say the earlier the better, but better late than never. There are some vices that pregnant women and women trying to conceive should avoid. These include alcohol, smoking, marijuana, and caffeine.

Alcohol

We've all heard the myth that a glass of red wine a day is okay to have when you're pregnant, but this couldn't be further from the truth. There is just no safe level of alcohol consumption during pregnancy, despite all the conflicting information you may find online or hear in passing. Alcohol should be absolutely avoided by expectant mothers and those attempting to conceive until after the baby is born.

Fetal alcohol spectrum disorders (FASD), are a group of developmental, emotional, mental, and physical problems and illnesses that can affect the fetus should the expectant mother decide to imbibe throughout the pregnancy. Similar to any liquid or food consumed by a pregnant woman, alcoholic beverages will pass to the fetus through the umbilical cord and into the placenta. So, if a pregnant woman drinks heavily, her high blood alcohol levels can prevent vital nutrients from reaching the baby, which is harmful for the baby's development. It takes around 2 hours for a fetus' blood alcohol level to be on par with that of its mother, and the alcohol ends up staying in its system for longer because their metabolisms are slower than ours. So, if one chooses to drink frequently or to excess, their fetus will be exposed to alcohol for longer.

That's why it's always better for women to quit drinking and abstain from it from the moment they suspect they're pregnant.

Can Alcohol Cause Birth Defects?

Birth defects are physical abnormalities that are present in the body before birth. They're caused by teratogens, which include alcohol.

Birth malformations caused by alcohol's impact on physical and structural development include:

- height and weight that are below average.

- issues with hearing and vision.

- bone, heart, and renal issues.

- small head circumference.

- abnormal facial features that might include:

    - a smooth ridge between the nose and upper lip.

    - an upturned nose.

    - a flat nasal bridge.

    - a thin upper lip.

Caffeine

Caffeine is a natural substance found in fruits, leaves, and seeds like cocoa beans and coffee beans. It also ends up in a lot of man-made foods like chocolate, ice cream, and the like.

There's no way to completely avoid it, but if you can keep your intake down to 200 milligrams per day, you'll be okay. It may sound far-fetched, but according to studies, more than 200 milligrams of caffeine per day while pregnant can cause harm. Caffeine consumption has been associated with a higher risk of miscarriage and low birth weight.

The precise amount of caffeine in a cup of coffee is difficult to determine because it can vary depending on the brand, preparation method, and cup size.

Here are some ways you can cut back on caffeine:

- Limit your coffee intake to a cup or two a day (be sure to pay attention to the size of the cup).

- Mix your regular coffee with some decaf.

- Start to phase out your regular coffee until you're only drinking decaf.

Keep in mind that green tea and other soft drinks also have caffeine. You can switch to decaffeinated versions. There are still trace amounts of caffeine, but nowhere near the amount that would be harmful to you and your baby.

You can still have chocolate in moderation, because the caffeine content in a chocolate bar varies from 5 to 30 milligrams.

Smoking

Smoking and pregnancy don't go together. Smoking during pregnancy is dangerous for both the mother and the unborn child. Nicotine, tar, and carbon monoxide are among the harmful chemicals found in cigarettes. Smoking greatly increases the chance of difficulties during pregnancy, some of which can be deadly.

Here are seven dangers one can encounter while smoking during pregnancy:

Birth Defects

Smoking increases the likelihood that a baby will be born with defects. Congenital cardiac abnormalities—abnormalities with the structure of the heart—and cleft lip and palate are among the most prevalent.

Ectopic pregnancy

See page. 37

Low birth weight

Smoking can contribute to low birth weight in newborns, but it goes beyond simply giving birth to a smaller baby. Other health issues and disabilities can occur too. Thankfully, the number of deaths caused by low birth weight has decreased tremendously because of medical advancements. However, it's still a severe condition, and it can lead to:

- delayed development

- hearing and vision impairment

- cerebral palsy

Miscarriage and stillbirth

Smoking increases the risk of miscarriages and stillbirths because cigarettes contain hazardous compounds that are harmful to babies.

Placental abruption

Smoking increases the risk of numerous placenta-related problems, the main one being placental abruption.

Placenta previa

See page. 94

Preterm labor

See page. 94

Marijuana

Marijuana is the most widely used illicit substance among pregnant women in the United States. A lot of pregnant women consider it a secure, all-natural cure for morning sickness, nausea, and vomiting. However, using marijuana while pregnant has significant, even fatal, risks.

Marijuana (even in small doses) has not been proven safe to use during pregnancy. The American Academy of Pediatrics issued its first set of official guidelines in 2018, recommending pregnant and breastfeeding women abstain from using marijuana since it poses risks to both mother and child.

Studies indicate that marijuana usage during pregnancy can result in:

- Low birth weight

- A higher chance of stillbirth

- Fetal growth restriction

- Preterm birth

- Ongoing brain development issues that affect behavior, learning, and memory

Narcotics: What Are the Effects in the Womb and After Birth?

Unfortunately, it's not uncommon for women of childbearing age to use illicit substances. Cocaine and other illegal drugs can have terrible effects on a fetus.

An expectant mom who takes illegal substances is at risk of so many other things. She's at risk of anemia, hepatitis, skin infections, blood infections, and heart infections. Over and above that, she is more vulnerable to developing STIs.

Everything a mother ingests gets transferred to the baby through the placenta, so any drugs she takes increase the likelihood of drug dependence in the unborn child.

The use of cocaine, methamphetamine, dextroamphetamine, methadone, and other opiates has been linked to stillbirth, preterm birth, placenta detachment, high blood pressure, and miscarriage. They also might cause withdrawal symptoms in newborns, like jitteriness, difficulty falling asleep, and feeding difficulties. Later on, they may experience issues with muscular tone and tremors. They are also more vulnerable to SIDS. Some symptoms linger for a few weeks, and these babies are more likely to have apnea and struggle to feed.

Mothers who use drugs during pregnancy are more likely to have low birth weight babies who might be more susceptible to:

- growth problems

- hyperactivity

- behavioral issues

- learning issues

A woman's chances of having a healthy baby increase if she stops using illicit drugs during the first trimester.

When the subject of pregnancy is brought up, the first thing that comes to mind is being more mindful about what you put into your body. Something we rarely talk about is our environment and how it needs to be healthy too. So…

Let's Talk Toxoplasma

Toxoplasma is a parasite that can be found in unwashed fruits and vegetables, raw or uncooked meat, soil, contaminated water, and anywhere that cat feces are present. Should you come into contact with it, you can develop toxoplasmosis, which is dangerous for you, and your unborn child.

Ways You Can Get It

- Consuming contaminated water.

- Using contaminated utensils or a cutting board that has come into contact with raw meat.

- Consuming undercooked or raw meat, or putting your hands in your mouth after handling uncooked meat.

- Accidentally consuming cat feces by touching your mouth after handling the litter box, touching soil, or anything else that's been in contact with it.

How It Affects You and Your Baby

Toxoplasmosis isn't always immediately detectable and can be hard to diagnose. People can be infected without having any noticeable symptoms, which means a pregnant woman could easily expose her fetus without even being aware of her condition. That's why it's so important to prevent it.

Symptoms include

- Headaches

- Swollen glands

- Muscle pain

- Fever

- A stiff neck

Visit a medical professional right away if you suffer from any of the aforementioned symptoms.

Toxoplasma in babies can cause blindness, intellectual impairment, and hearing damage. Even years after birth, some children may experience difficulties with their eyes or brains.

Babies born with the infection may also need years of specialized care, like special education and ophthalmology care.

In order to lessen the impact of the parasite, it's crucial to identify and treat the infection as soon as possible.

How You Can Prevent It

Cook

- Don't taste-test meat until it's cooked.

- Always make sure the meat is completely cooked. It should be cooked internally to a temperature of 160° F (71° C). To check, use a food thermometer.

Clean

- After handling raw meat, cat litter, soil, or unwashed produce, wash your hands with soap and warm water.

- Always wash your utensils and cutting board with warm, soapy water after use.

- All fruits and vegetables should be thoroughly washed and/or peeled before consumption.

Separate

- Separate raw meat from the other food in your fridge. Also, keep raw meat away when you're handling or preparing other food.

Always make sure that any water you consume has been treated. Should you travel to a less developed country while you're pregnant, be vigilant and mindful, or just stick to bottled water.

If you have a cat, you don't have to get rid of it. Just bear in mind that toxoplasma infects virtually all cats that spend any time outdoors. They get it by consuming contaminated raw meat or small animals. The parasite is subsequently spread via the cat's droppings. A pregnant woman might not be aware that her cat has it because toxoplasma doesn't make cats appear ill.

Here are some tips you can follow to prevent or lessen the chances of contracting it from your cat:

- Avoid stray cats (especially kittens).

- Feed your cat dry or canned food; avoid letting them near raw meat.

- Have someone else change the litter box if at all possible. If you must clean it, put on disposable gloves and then thoroughly wash your hands with warm water and soap.

- The parasite takes one to five days to become contagious, so changing your litter box daily can help prevent contraction.

- Wear gloves when tending your garden in case there's any excrement in the soil. When you're done, wash your hands.

Now that your environment is safe for YOU, let's see how you can ensure that your body is a safe environment for babies.

Keeping Fit While Pregnant

For some, pregnancy's a breeze. For others, it's months of discomfort and feeling like you're no longer in charge of your body. Exercising regularly can offset some of that discomfort and keep you healthy throughout your pregnancy. It can also minimize some common aches, pains, and exhaustion. Exercise also helps alleviate stress, lessens your chances of developing gestational diabetes, and helps you build the endurance you need for labor and delivery.

If you exercised regularly before pregnancy, you can keep it up, just at a slower rate, and with less intensity. Always listen to your body and do what you can handle. If you didn't previously exercise, you can speak to your doctor about starting a nice and safe regimen. A good place to start would be about 30 minutes of mild to moderate exercise once daily. Keep in mind that exercise doesn't have to be taxing on the body to be beneficial.

Exercise Tips

- Drink plenty of fluids, especially water.

- Never work out without warming up beforehand, and always cool down afterward.

- Should you decide to join a class, make sure the instructor has experience with pregnant women.

- Try and exercise daily; even a walk is okay. Avoid strenuous exercise, especially in the heat.

- Given that water will sustain your increasing weight, you might want to give swimming a try. Aqua-natal sessions are offered at a few local swimming facilities with trained instructors. Find a pool in your area.

- Do your best to avoid exercises where there's a possibility you'll fall. For example, horse riding or cycling.

Exercises to Avoid

- After 16 weeks, avoid lying flat on your back for prolonged periods since the pressure from your bump on the main blood vessel transporting blood to your heart can cause you to feel dizzy.

- Avoid engaging in contact sports like kickboxing, martial arts, or squash, where there is a chance of getting hit.

- Avoid scuba diving because your baby won't be protected against gas embolism (gas bubbles in the bloodstream) and decompression sickness.

- Never exercise at 2500 meters above sea level because altitude sickness is a concern for both you and the baby.

Who Shouldn't Exercise While Pregnant?

If you have a preexisting condition like diabetes or asthma, exercise is not recommended. Exercise can also be harmful when you've got pregnancy-related conditions like:

- A weak cervix

- Continual or imminent miscarriage

- Low placenta

- Past preterm births or a history of premature labor

Which Exercises Are Safe?

As long as you work out carefully and don't overdo it, most exercises are safe to do while pregnant.

Here's a list of workouts you can incorporate into your routine. They will strengthen your muscles enough to help you carry any added weight. They'll also strengthen your joints, increase circulation, relieve back pain, and generally make you feel good.

Abdominal Exercise

As your pregnancy progresses, you may notice a dip in your lower back deepening, which can cause back pain. These exercises can help with that while strengthening your abdominal muscles:

- Get onto all fours and keep your back straight, by lifting your abdominals and placing your hands beneath your shoulders with your fingers pointing forward.

- Curl your trunk and let your head softly relax forward while contracting your abdominal muscles and raising your back towards the ceiling. Try not to let your elbows lock.

- Hold for a brief moment before returning gradually to the box position.

- Keep in mind that your back should always return to its natural, straight position.

- Make your muscles work hard and carefully move your back as you repeat this motion ten times slowly and methodically.

- Only move your back in a way that's comfortable, don't strain it.

Pelvic Floor Exercises

The pelvic floor is made up of layers of muscles that extend from the pubic bone to the tailbone. It's shaped like a hammock. Our pelvic floor muscles get put under a lot of strain while we're pregnant and once we've given birth.

If your pelvic floor becomes weak, urine can escape if you cough or sneeze. It's called "stress incontinence," and there's nothing to be embarrassed about. It happens to a lot of women after birth.

Exercises that target the pelvic floor can help you develop these muscles. This aids in preventing or reducing postpartum stress incontinence. Even if you're young and don't currently experience stress incontinence, every pregnant woman should do it.

- Close up your bottom, like you're trying to hold it in a while using the restroom.

- Draw in your urethra like you're stopping the flow of pee while also drawing in your vagina like you're grasping a tampon.

- Perform this exercise quickly at first, immediately contracting and relaxing the muscles.

- Slow it down by holding the contractions for up to ten seconds at a time.

- Try to do three sets of eight daily. A good rule of thumb is to do it before or after every meal.

- For even better results, do pelvic floor exercises before and during a cough or sneeze.

Pelvic Tilt Exercises

- Stand, and put your bottom and shoulders up against a wall.

- Soften your knees.

- Draw your belly button toward your spine so that your back is completely straight, then release after 4 seconds of holding.

- Do this repeatedly, up to ten times.

Vitamins and Supplements

We get most of the vitamins we need from the food we eat, but should there be a deficit, we can supplement our intake with herbal supplements, fish oil capsules, single minerals, and multivitamins.

In order for your baby to grow and develop at a healthy rate, you need to be sure you're getting good amounts of all the nutrients you need.

In pregnancy, our need for certain nutrients increases to account for ourselves and the baby. These include folate, iodine, iron, vitamins B and D, and protein.

- Folate is vital. It prevents neural tube defects, especially when taken very early in the pregnancy.

- Iodine aids in the development of the brain and the nervous system.

- Iron helps prevent low birth weight in the baby and anemia in the mother.

- Vitamins B and D assist with the growth of the baby's skeleton and nervous system. Adding vitamin C to the mix will help you and your baby better absorb iron from your diet.

Should You Be Taking Supplements?

All pregnant women are advised to take vitamin D, iron, and folic acid supplements. All the other vitamins you need should ideally come from your diet, especially if it's a healthy one. Some pregnant women, however, do need to supplement more than the three main vitamins as well.

Your doctor may recommend more supplements for you if:

- You're vegan/vegetarian and don't get enough vitamin B12.

- You can't get enough calcium from dairy or other calcium-rich foods.

- You lack iron.

- If you eat little to no seafood and aren't getting enough omega-3 fatty acids.

Multivitamins designed for pregnant women are a welcome addition to your new routine. Keep in mind that they don't serve as a replacement for a balanced diet. It's important to keep your diet healthy and nutrient-dense even if you're taking multivitamins.

Each vitamin is only slightly necessary for your body, and larger amounts are not always advised. Overindulging has negative effects. For instance, taking excessive amounts of vitamins A, C, or E can be harmful. So, there's no need to supplement those vitamins during pregnancy. You should also stay away from foods like liver and its byproducts because they're extremely high in vitamin A.

Diet

Everything you eat and drink while you're pregnant should support your health and provide the nutrients your unborn child needs to grow and develop. That means your diet should be balanced, nutrient-dense, and low in salt, sugar, and saturated fats.

Gaining weight during pregnancy is normal, but doing so at the expense of your health or the health of your baby puts you at greater risk of experiencing complications.

Your pre-pregnancy weight affects how much weight you can gain safely. There is evidence to support using BMI as a benchmark when determining the ideal weight gain during pregnancy.

A balanced diet is more than enough for you to get all the nutrients you need, but some foods have higher amounts of specific nutrients that are especially important during pregnancy.

We've done all this talking about a balanced diet, but we haven't specified exactly what that is.

What Constitutes a Balanced Diet?

A balanced diet is a wide variety of nutrient-dense foods from the five food groups, and lots and lots of water:

1. Fruit

2. Legumes and vegetables

3. Cereals and wholegrains

4. Dairy

5. Lean meats

Nobody's perfect. There'll be days where you're on your best behavior and eating all the right things, and there'll be days where you may treat yourself a little more than usual. Cravings will definitely make it harder to stay away from sugars and saturated fats.

There's an old theory that cravings are an indicator of vitamin deficiencies in a pregnant mother's diet. There isn't much evidence to support this because our tastes change so much when we're pregnant. We start to dislike things we liked and begin to like things we disliked.

With everything happening in our bodies and our hormones going haywire, we may also start to develop food aversions. If you experience unbearable morning sickness, eat whatever you can stomach and contact a medical professional if you start to get worried.

Which Foods Should I Avoid?

Some foods contain harmful bacteria or parasites that could contribute to serious difficulties for the unborn child and raise the possibility of miscarriage. Below is a list of the types of foods to avoid while pregnant:

Seafood High in Mercury

Seafood is pretty iffy. On the one hand, it's a great source of omega-3 fatty acids, which are amazing for a baby's brain development, and on the other, some forms of seafood have so much mercury in them that they could threaten your baby's nervous system.

The likelihood of a fish containing more mercury increases with size and age. The Food and Drug Administration (FDA) recommends that you stay away from:

- Tilefish

- Swordfish

- Shark

- Orange roughy

- Marlin

- King mackerel

- Bigeye tuna

Worry not; there is seafood out there with very small concentrations of mercury that is safe to eat and is a good source of protein. You can have two to three servings per week of:

- Trout

- Tilapia

- Shrimp

- Shad

- Sardines

- Salmon

- Pollock

- Pacific Oysters

- Light canned tuna

- Herring

- Cod

- Catfish

- Anchovies

Raw, Undercooked, or Contaminated Seafood

- Don't eat raw fish or shellfish. This includes ceviche, raw oysters, scallops, sashimi, sushi, and clams.

- Steer clear of raw, refrigerated seafood. This includes: nova-style seafood; lox; kippers; jerky; or smoked foods. You can have smoked seafood if it's part of another dish or if it's canned.

- Always look at fish advisories for your area, especially if you're eating local fish.

- Cook seafood thoroughly. Fish should be cooked to a temperature of 145°F. Consider your food cooked when it flakes and becomes opaque all throughout. Cook lobster, scallops, and shrimp until they are milky white. And oysters, mussels, and clams should be cooked until their shells open. Throw the ones that don't open away.

Undercooked Meat, Poultry, and Eggs

In order to avoid foodborne illness:

- Use a meat thermometer to make sure that everything is fully cooked and ready to eat.

- Avoid eating hot dogs and luncheon meats altogether, or cook them to a boiling temperature. They may be sources of listeria infections.

- Keep chilled pateo and meat spreads to a minimum. Canned and shelf-stable spreads are okay.

- Eggs should be cooked until the yolks and whites are set because raw eggs contain potentially dangerous bacteria. Steer clear of anything made with partially cooked eggs. This includes wet batter, eggnog, hollandaise sauce, or Caesar salad dressing.

Unpasteurized Foods

Unpasteurized milk products can lead to foodborne illness. Soft cheeses like brie, blue cheese, and feta shouldn't be consumed unless they're prepared from pasteurized milk or are clearly labeled as such. Avoid unpasteurized juices too.

Low-fat dairy products are the safer option. This includes: cottage cheese, mozzarella, and skim milk.

Unwashed Fruits and Veggies

All raw fruits and vegetables should be thoroughly washed to get rid of any dangerous bacteria. Steer clear of raw sprouts. This includes: mung bean, alfalfa, clover, and radish. When you eat sprouts, ensure that they're properly cooked.

Food Prep

If ever there was a time to be fussy about food safety, it was during pregnancy. Do so prudently, because contaminated food is the leading cause of food poisoning. Sometimes it's easy to spot when food smells or looks different. But sometimes it's less obvious, so to be on the safe side, you should always:

- Defrost your meat in the microwave.

- Wash your hands before cooking and again before eating.

- Have separate cutting boards for meat and veggies.

- Change dishcloths often, because once there's a smell, it's probably contaminated.

- Cook and reheat your meat thoroughly; make sure it's at least 140°F and steaming when you reheat.

Recommended Serving Size

Food Group	Servings per Day
Fruit	2
Legumes and vegetables	5
Cereals and whole grains	8
Dairy	3.5
Lean meats	3.5

(Healthdirect Australia, 2022)

Medication During Pregnancy

A lot of medications say "Not safe for pregnant or lactating women" on the packaging, so it's hard for us to know what we can and can't take. Pregnant women are not typically used in drug studies because researchers are concerned about the effects on unborn babies. There are some medications that have been around for so long that doctors can attest to their safety for pregnant women.

It's generally safe to take the following:

Over-the-counter medication

- Acetaminophen for pain and fever (like Tylenol)

- Certain antihistamines, like loratadine and diphenhydramine (like Claritin and Benadryl)

Prescription medication

- Hypertension medication

- Asthma medication

- Antidepressants

- Penicillin and other antibiotics

- HIV medication

Speaking of medication, who better to advise you than your doctor? Let's look at your first visit with them and what that may be like.

First Antenatal Visit—What to Expect—Who Will I Meet?

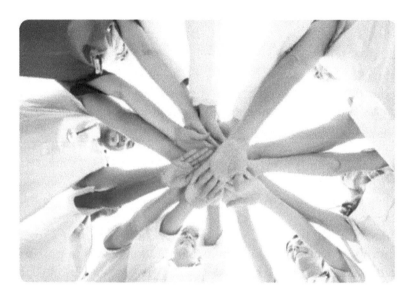

Your first visit is basically for you to find out how far along you actually are, and for your doctor to get to know about your medical history up until this point. The doctor will also run a series of standard tests just to make sure you and baby are okay.

Some things your doctor might ask about:

- Your gynecological history, any past pregnancies, and your last menstrual cycle.

- Your medical histories, both personal and familial.

- Exposure to potentially harmful substances.

- Any medication you're taking: pharmaceutical and homeopathic.

- Your lifestyle.

- Whether you've traveled in the last six months.

Your doctor will then perform a physical exam that includes a breast and pelvic exam. Depending on your general health, you might need tests of your thyroid, lungs, and heart. The doctor will also calculate your BMI to find out how much weight you need to gain for a safe pregnancy.

Then, in order to get your estimated due date, they will use the beginning of your last period, plus seven days, then go back three months. It will be roughly 40 weeks after the first day of your most recent period. Estimating the due date is important because it allows medical personnel to properly monitor your progress and the baby's growth.

Your due date doesn't necessarily indicate when you'll give birth. Very few women actually go into labor on their due date.

The blood tests your doctor may order include the following:

- A test to determine blood type

- A test to measure your hemoglobin

- A test to check your immunity levels

- A test to detect exposure to infection

Rh Factor: Why Will I Be Tested? What Happens if It's Positive?

Your blood type's Rh factor isn't an issue in general, but being Rh-negative is a problem if your baby is Rh-positive. Your body will produce antibodies that could harm your baby's red blood cells if your blood types mix. Your baby can get anemia and possibly develop other issues as a result of this.

Each person belongs to one of the four main blood types: A, B, AB, or O. The types of antigens on blood cells determine blood types. Antigens are proteins located on the surface of blood cells that can trigger reactions in the immune system. The Rh factor is one of those proteins. Rh-positive individuals have the Rh factor, and Rh-negative people don't.

If you turn out to be Rh-negative while your baby is positive, the antibodies you produce can affect your baby. Your body may react as though you were allergic to the baby if a small amount of the baby's blood mixes with yours. As a result of your increased sensitivity, your antibodies are now able to cross the placenta and target the blood of your unborn child. Once they start to break the baby's red blood cells down, it leads to anemia. This specific type of anemia is called "hemolytic disease" or "hemolytic anemia." It has the potential to harm the fetus' brain, cause major illness, or kill them.

If you go for all your prenatal checkups and get all your blood tests; doctors can find this out in time and intervene. If your body hasn't yet produced the antibodies, the doctor can inject you with Rh immunoglobulin and prevent the development of antibodies.

If you've already developed them, Rh immunoglobulin is ineffective. All the doctors can do is closely monitor yours and the baby's conditions until you give birth. If the baby is delivered on time, they may receive a blood transfusion to replace the sick blood cells with healthy ones. In more extreme situations, the baby could need to be delivered early or get transfusions while still in utero.

Hepatitis B: Why Will I Be Tested?

An estimated 73,000 people contract the viral illness hepatitis B each year. It's carried by about 1,250,000 people in the United States. About 30% of those affected will not show symptoms, but symptoms include: (*Hepatitis B explained*, 2019)

- abdominal pain

- fatigue

- jaundice

- nausea

- vomiting

- reduced appetite

There is no treatment for it, so once you get it, you're infected for the rest of your life. It can lead to serious liver damage. Liver failure and liver cancer claim the lives of about 5,000 people annually.

Hepatitis B is spread through sexual activity, from mother to child, from contact with contaminated blood, and via IV drug use.

You can avoid it by abstain from unprotected sex, being in a monogamous relationship, and refraining from injecting narcotics. There is a vaccine, and that's by far the best way to prevent this illness.

Sickle Cell, Why Test?

Sickle cell disease is a congenital genetic disorder characterized by defective hemoglobin. It prevents the red blood cells' hemoglobin from carrying oxygen. Sickle cells have a propensity to cluster, obstructing tiny blood vessels and resulting in painful and detrimental complications. Children who inherit two sickle cell genes—one from each parent—get it. A person who has SCD can pass the trait on to their children.

Sickle cell trait is not a disease, but a gene that one inherits from a parent. SCT patients typically don't experience any SCD symptoms and have normal lives, but they can pass the sickle cell gene to their offspring as well.

As soon as a woman decides she'd like to get pregnant, she, along with her partner, should get tested for SCT. Most hospitals and medical facilities offer testing, as do many community-based organizations and regional health departments. A genetic counselor can offer further information and further explore the dangers to their children if a woman or her spouse has SCT.

What Are the Odds?

When both parents have SCT, there is a 25% probability that each pregnancy will result in a child with SCD.

When both parents have SCT, there is a 50% probability that each pregnancy will result in a child with SCT.

(CDC, n.d.)

Can a Woman Have SCD and a Healthy Pregnancy?

A woman with SCD can have a healthy pregnancy if she receives early prenatal care and has close supervision throughout her pregnancy.

Pregnant women with SCD are, however, more prone to experiencing issues that could harm both their health and the health of their unborn child. They should visit their obstetrician, hematologist, or general care physician frequently.

SCD can worsen during pregnancy, so the bouts of pain will be more frequent.

There's also a higher chance of preterm labor and low birth weight in babies born to pregnant women with SCD.

Your Baby's Development

POPPY SEED

Assuming you've taken a pregnancy test because you've missed your period, you're four weeks along.

Four weeks? That probably doesn't sound right, because you likely conceived two or three weeks ago. We start measuring pregnancy from the first day of your last menstrual cycle, so technically, you're four weeks long.

Your body is starting to build the placenta and amniotic sac.

You may experience abdominal discomfort and sore breasts as the group of cells that will eventually form your baby penetrates the lining of your uterus. You may also experience some implantation bleeding. If you're not showing any symptoms, that's normal too.

Your baby is as tiny as a poppy seed at the moment. They are still a ball of cells, but they've managed to find a nice, comfy spot in your uterus and set up shop. After about 6–10 days, the ball starts dividing some more and ends up as two bundles of cells. The inner bundle of cells will become your baby, while the outer bundle will become the placenta. This is the time when your baby graduates from being a blastocyst to an embryo.

The embryo is tiny, but mighty. It has three layers that form the building blocks for your little baby:

- **The endoderm**: The innermost layer that will eventually become the liver, lungs, and digestive system.

- **The mesoderm**: The middle layer that will eventually become the heart, kidneys, bones, muscles, and sex organs.

- **The ectoderm**: The outermost layer that will eventually become the brain, skin, nervous system, eyes, and hair.

Judging by the amount of information here, a lot can happen in a month. Let's see what happens in the next one.

Chapter 2: Month Two

You've taken a pregnancy test, you've seen the positive sign, and now that it's confirmed…

You May Be Experiencing…

- **Fatigue**: During the first trimester of pregnancy, progesterone levels rise, which may cause you to feel sleepier or more exhausted than usual.

- **Frequent urination**: Your kidneys create extra fluid because they have to work harder during pregnancy since your blood volume increases. That means you'll be in the loo quite often.

- **Sensitive breasts**: Your breasts will most probably feel painful and uncomfortable when you first get pregnant. But this usually goes away as your body becomes used to the change in hormones.

- **Nausea and/or vomiting**: After a missed period, nausea is the most obvious sign of pregnancy. Some women only experience it within the first three months, others have it throughout the entire pregnancy.

- **Bloating**: Pregnancy hormones tend to make you feel bloated. You could mistake the bloating for a sign of PMS.

- **Cramping**: You may experience some uterine cramping due to all the changes in your hormonal balance.

- **Spotting**: Some women mistake spotting for a period, but it's lighter and is a good indicator that one is pregnant.

Prenatal Tests: Why They're So Important

Pregnancy is nine months of pure anticipation (and sometimes anxiety). You wake up every day wondering what your baby's going to look like, who they'll grow up to be, and most importantly, whether they'll come out with ten fingers and toes. The truth is, most babies are born healthy, but it's okay to be concerned. You have every right to do all that you can to find out whether your baby will be healthy and what steps you can take should you find out they won't be, and that's where prenatal testing comes in. The two main types are:

Screening tests: Many birth defects and genetic illnesses can be detected during prenatal screening tests. You'll also find out the likelihood of your baby having them. They come in the form of blood tests, a special ultrasound, and prenatal cell-free DNA screening. These tests are usually concluded by the second trimester. Keep in mind that they're unable to make a definitive diagnosis; they can just indicate risk. Should your doctor pick up any risk factors, you'll be scheduled for a diagnostic test as soon as possible.

Diagnostic tests: If you've had a screening test done and your age, family history, or medical history puts you at elevated risk of delivering a baby with a genetic condition, the only way to get a definitive diagnosis is via a diagnostic test. They can be invasive. The two main ones are amniocentesis and chorionic villus sampling. They have the potential to cause miscarriages.

Miscarriage

Another word for miscarriage is *spontaneous abortion.* The majority of miscarriages are unavoidable and happen when the fetus stops developing. These things happen, and nine times out of ten, they're out of our hands.

There are different types of miscarriage, namely:

Missed miscarriage: In these cases, the mother is usually unaware that a miscarriage has occurred. It can only be confirmed if the fetus is found to be without a heartbeat on an ultrasound.

Complete miscarriage: This one is obvious because there will be bleeding and the fetal tissue will pass through you. In this case, the pregnancy is completely over and your uterus is empty.

Threatened miscarriage: Your cervix remains closed, but you'll experience bleeding and have cramps in your pelvis. There usually aren't any further complications, and the pregnancy continues as normal. But for the remainder of your pregnancy, your obstetrician may keep a closer eye on you.

Inevitable miscarriage: Your cervix opens, you dilate, and you possibly leak blood and some amniotic fluid. There are high chances of miscarrying completely.

Recurrent miscarriage: Three successive miscarriages. It affects only 1% of expectant mothers.

Ectopic Pregnancy

Ectopic pregnancies usually occur in the fallopian tube; you may also know them as tubal pregnancies. But sometimes they happen in other parts of the body, like the abdominal cavity, the cervix, or the ovary. These types of pregnancies cannot develop properly because the fertilized egg can't survive anywhere other than the womb. If left untreated, the expanding tissue may result in a life-threatening hemorrhage.

Symptoms include:

- **Normal pregnancy symptoms**: In the beginning, there will be no warning signs. Everything will feel normal. A missed period, nausea, etc.

- **Vaginal bleeding and pelvic pain**: The initial warning signs are light vaginal bleeding and pelvic pain. Should your fallopian tube bleed, your shoulders could ache, and you may feel the need to urinate frequently. It all depends on which nerves become inflamed and where the blood gathers.

- **A ruptured tube**: The fallopian tube could burst if the fertilized egg is left there long enough to start growing. This then leads to bleeding in the abdomen and then lightheadedness, shock, and fainting.

Should you experience any or all of the above symptoms, contact your doctor immediately.

Multiples?

The only surefire way to know whether or not you're having multiples is via ultrasound, but there are some little telltale signs that might be clues that you've got more than one bun in the oven.

Several women who've been pregnant with twins say that even before they were certain, they had a hunch or felt they were. For others, the news comes as a great shock.

Here are some signs that seem to have popped up in lots of pregnancies:

- **Measuring ahead**: Although some women who are carrying twins claim to start showing earlier, the exact time depends on the individual and the pregnancy. Many women start to show sooner if it's their second pregnancy.

- **Increased weight gain**: Another warning sign that might not surface until later in your pregnancy. Weight gain in your first trimester of pregnancy is probably going to be minimal. If you notice rapid weight gain in the first trimester, contact your OB/GYN to discuss the possible reasons

- **Early movement**: It's possible to feel movement a little bit earlier with two or more infants than with just one, but it's still likely to happen in the second trimester as well.

In 2018, there were 32.6 twins for every 1,000 live births, according to the CDC. The number of twin births each year is influenced by a wide range of factors. The likelihood of having twins can be increased by elements like genetics, age, and fertility treatments.

While having multiples is fantastic, there are certain risks involved. It's crucial to pay attention to your health and seek prenatal care.

Choosing Your Birth Plan

Labor and delivery seldom go according to plan, but it's normal to want some control over how you bring your child into this world. It's a really big deal, it's scary, and it's best to be as prepared as humanly possible.

A birth plan can help manage your expectations and pave the way for a seamless experience despite the overwhelming amount of decisions to be made.

Even though your plans may change as you go, mapping out your ideal labor and delivery will help you make important choices that will help your support team keep you and your unborn child safe and comfortable.

If you're unsure of your birth plan, here's a thorough list of questions that can nudge you in the right direction:

Environment

1. Do you want to give birth at home, in a hospital, or at a birthing center?

2. Would you like a specific kind of lighting?

3. Would you like photography or videography?

4. Would you like music playing in the room?

5. Would you like to be fully dressed?

People

1. Who will look after you while you are in labor?

2. Would you like a birthing coach?

3. Who is permitted to be present during the birth or to visit immediately after?

4. Would you allow medical students to be present if you gave birth in a teaching hospital?

Upon arrival

1. Would you prefer to have the hair on your pubic region shaved? Many hospitals no longer allow prenatal shaving, but it wouldn't hurt to ask.

2. What are your thoughts on getting an enema? Like shaving, they're no longer commonplace. But it wouldn't hurt to find out whether it's an expectation.

3. Are you okay with getting a routine IV?

4. Are you allowed to watch your cesarean section by mirror?

5. Would you like to eat and drink during labor? This all depends on your procedure and how everything goes on the day, but you can inquire about the policies.

Interventions

1. Would you like fetal monitoring?

2. What's your take on internal and external exams?

3. What are your feelings on induced labor and artificial membrane rupturing?

4. Is an episiotomy welcome or unwelcome?

5. Are you open to forceps and vacuum extraction?

6. Do you have any specific preferences or worries regarding having a C-section?

7. When or under what conditions would you think about having any of the above procedures?

Labor and delivery

1. Which type of pain management would you prefer— medical or natural?

2. Will you be active while giving birth? If so, how active?

3. Would you like a shower or a bath while in labor?

4. Is there a specific type of food you'd like during labor?

5. How long can you wait before cutting the umbilical cord?

6. Who would you like to cut the cord?

7. How soon and for how long will you and your partner be able to interact with the baby after birth?

8. How soon should you feed your baby after birth?

Postpartum

1. Will the baby remain in your care or in the nursery?

2. Where will your partner and other children stay while you're away?

3. Will you breastfeed or bottle-feed? Will you need assistance with either?

4. Will you consent to the baby having supplemental bottle-feeds?

5. Should you give the baby a pacifier?

6. Who will give the baby their first bath? Would you need help doing it?

7. Will you have the child circumcised? If so, when and by whom?

8. What are the rules of the NICU should your baby be admitted?

Going home

1. Will you be using a car seat?

2. Do you have pre-arranged transportation to get you home?

3. Should you prepare the first few family dinners in advance for when you get home?

4. Do you need a strategy for pet-proofing your baby's nursery or sleeping area?

5. Do you require company while you get settled at home?

Your Baby's Development

BEANS

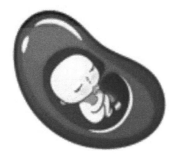

So, you may not be showing, but it's likely that your clothing is feeling a bit snug. That's because by month two, your uterus—which is typically the size of a fist—has expanded to the size of a giant grapefruit.

In the grand scheme of things, that's pretty small. So, even if you probably don't appear pregnant on the outside, you surely do on the inside.

By now, the baby is around 1/2 to 2/3 of an inch long and is about the size of a kidney bean. The baby is growing by a millimeter everyday and is developing its lips, nose, and eyelids.

The bulk of your baby is actually its head, where the brain is forming and building at an astonishing rate. The nerve cells are proliferating and connecting to create a neural network that will one day be able to pass messages from the brain to the body.

Your baby's limbs are bulking up and getting longer, thanks to their developing bones and cartilage. They're also close to developing joints, so there will eventually be elbows, shoulders, and knees to look forward to. The umbilical cord is starting to make an appearance, and get this, the intestines are inside it. They will migrate into the body when the time is right.

It's still early days, but things are getting serious. Now is a better time than any to try and start finding out if everything is going according to plan.

Chapter 3: Month Three

Emotions in Trimester One

Most of us will spend the majority of our pregnancies worrying, but nothing compares to the anxiety we might feel in the first trimester. Once month three is over, there's a bit of reprieve because that's known as the "safe zone," where the chance of miscarriage is significantly reduced.

Now, it's everything else as well. You worry about your future child's health, the delivery process, your connections with friends and family, how having a baby will impact those relationships, and the financial strain of adding to your family. These concerns are all reasonable, and a certain level of anxiety is actually protective for us. It's there to push us so we can see ourselves through different phases of our lives.

Coping With Mood Swings

Your fast-changing hormones, particularly estrogen and progesterone, are a major contributing factor to mood swings throughout pregnancy. In the first 12 weeks, your estrogen levels rise by more than 100 times.

Estrogen and serotonin (the *happy* hormone) go hand in hand. Even though serotonin boosts feelings of happiness, it's not a shortcut to happiness. So all the imbalances and variations in that neurotransmitter (serotonin) can lead to emotional dysregulation.

Progesterone levels also rise quickly, particularly in the first three months. Progesterone is linked to relaxation, whereas estrogen is linked to energy (and too much of it is linked to neurotic energy).

Relaxing hormones sound appealing, but some progesterone can cause *too much* relaxation. It can lead to lethargy and sometimes even feelings of sadness. It's actually what makes you cry at the sight of seemingly normal things. It's no wonder you're so up and down. You've got estrogen making you excitable and progesterone making you teary.

Should your mood swings become unmanageable or sway more towards feelings of depression, consult your GP or healthcare professional. Getting in front of it before it gets bad will really help. You can look for support groups in your area or online.

First Trimester Mood Swings

Besides hormones, the physical changes of pregnancy can cause emotional distress. The main one is nausea. The faintest hunger pangs or the aroma of food cooking can cause nausea and perhaps vomiting. The urge to puke at inopportune times may cause you to feel anxious.

You may also start to feel anxious because you don't know when you'll start to feel sick, and there's always the threat of passing out in public or without warning. Another symptom that contributes to mood swings is fatigue. When you're exhausted, it can be hard to function well emotionally, and because you'll experience extreme fatigue in the first couple of months, you're more likely to feel dysregulated a lot of the time.

Last but not least, women who have lost pregnancies before may worry that it'll happen again because of the higher chances of miscarriage in the first three months.

With all these changes happening, it's easy to feel like you're not in control of a lot of things. You may want to do some of the things you used to do—the things that could help you feel *normal*.

Grooming is one of those things. It's okay to wax, dye your hair, use fake tan, and get a massage as long as you do so safely. You might want to wait until you're at least in your second trimester before attempting these things.

So, what can't you do?

Botox: Is It Okay?

Botox is the brand name, despite the widespread misunderstanding that all cosmetic neurotoxins are Botox. There are other neurotoxins that are also injected to reduce wrinkles and fine lines in a similar way. They consist of Xeomin, Jeauveau, and Dysport.

Botox is classified as being in the pregnancy category X, which means it's unsafe to use while pregnant. When a drug or a treatment has dangers that far outweigh the benefits, the FDA classes it under X. There is also evidence of fetal abnormalities associated with Botox.

Since the risks far outweigh the benefits, it's best to reschedule your Botox appointment after you've given birth.

Despite our best efforts, we can never fully prepare for all of life's tiny surprises. What if you already had Botox and then discovered you were pregnant? Your initial reaction can be one of dread, which is understandable. No adverse effects have been documented in studies on pregnant women who received Botox injections before discovering they were pregnant. It's unlikely to cause problems because it has very limited bioavailability in the bloodstream. If you find yourself in this situation, you can breathe; it's unlikely that anything bad will happen, but you should contact your doctor just in case.

Your Baby's Development

LIME

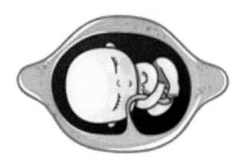

Your uterus, which is still roughly the size of a big grapefruit, starts to move from the bottom of your pelvis to the front and center of your abdomen.

If you're lucky, this will stop you from having to urinate all the time.

Some of the early pregnancy symptoms, like nausea, painful breasts and nipples, food aversions, and fatigue, are also expected to lessen considerably now that you're approaching the end of your first trimester. Your digestive system is starting to slow down now, so you'll absorb more nutrients, but you'll probably also experience bloating, gas, and constipation.

A lot has happened in the past month. Baby has doubled in size, measuring two to two and a quarter inches. The size of a small lime. All of the baby's vital organs and key body systems are fully formed. The brain structure is also complete, so brain matter will start to grow as the weeks' progress. The thyroid is fully functional, the pituitary gland has started producing hormones, and the pancreas is producing insulin. Lastly, a baby's bone marrow is starting to produce white blood cells to protect them against infection, and the muscles in their digestive tract are starting to contract so they'll be able to process food once they're born.

You should be able to hear your baby's heartbeat at your 12-week checkup, so you've got something really exciting to look forward to.

TRIMESTER 2:

The Honeymoon Period

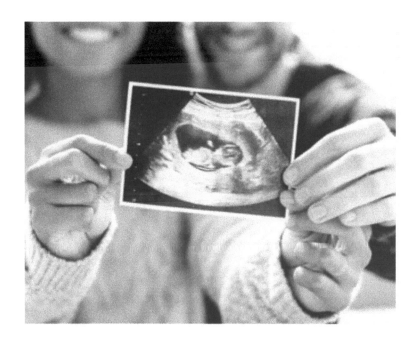

Chapter 4: Month Four

Emotions in the Second Trimester

The second trimester is often referred to as the "honeymoon" period. Although they are fluctuating far less than they were during the first three months, hormones are still fluctuating. Most women report having more energy and experiencing less morning sickness than before.

It's more comfortable, but it's not without its triggers. The main one being the changes in the body. In trimester one, you can get away with wearing your old clothes and essentially *hiding* your pregnancy. But in trimester two, you start to show, and you have to start considering maternity wear and sharing the news with people. Some women experience excitement at their physical changes. Some, though, may experience anxiety. This is especially true for women who've struggled with their body image

Other emotional anguish you may experience could be due to prenatal testing throughout the second trimester. When recommended, amniocentesis is typically performed early in the second trimester. You could feel anxious while deciding whether to get tests done or not, and then start stressing over the results and what they might reveal.

It's not all negative, though. Some women report a spike in libido. This may be a result of their physical health beginning to improve as well as increased blood supply to the pelvic area.

Figuring Out Your Ideal Weight

We gain weight to ensure we have enough nutrients for the fetus' development and to store enough nutrients to get ready for breastfeeding. Weight gain is completely normal, and needed during pregnancy, but research has revealed that specific weight gain ranges depending on BMI have better overall effects on the expectant mom and her baby.

The rule of thumb is to gain one to four pounds in the first trimester and then a pound every week thereafter. This can be done by eating an extra 300 calories per day.

Here is the recommended weight gain range:

Pregnancy BMI	Category	Total Weight Gain Range	Total Weight Gain Range for Pregnancy with Twins
<18.5	Under weight	28–40 lbs	
18.5–24.9	Normal weight	25–35 lbs	37–54 lbs
25.0–29.9	Overweight	15–35 lbs	31–50 lbs
≥ 30	Obese	11–20 lbs	25–42 lbs

(*Pregnancy Weight Gain Calculator*, 2009)

Potential Complications of Suboptimal Weight Gain

Both inadequate and excessive weight gain during pregnancy have their drawbacks. Inadequate weight gain can endanger the fetus' health and result in preterm labor or premature birth. Excessive weight gain can complicate labor, result in larger than normal babies, cause postpartum weight retention, and raise the chance that you'll have an emergency C-section.

Heartburn

When you're pregnant, the rise in progesterone causes several parts of your body to relax, so the lower esophageal sphincter (LES) fails to close properly, and the acid is able to move up into your esophagus.

Other causes include:

- **Changes in hormone levels**: Throughout pregnancy, your hormone levels fluctuate, which impacts how you absorb and digest food. Your digestive tract slows down, then food moves slowly, resulting in bloating and heartburn.

- **Uterus enlargement**: Your uterus grows bigger as your child develops, so all the organs surrounding it (including the stomach) become constricted. This ends up forcing stomach acid into your esophagus.

For relief from heartburn, you can eat yogurt or drink milk. Warm your milk and add a teaspoon of honey to it.

Over-the-counter antacids tend to be high in salt, and that could make you retain water. Several of them also include aluminum, which is unsafe during pregnancy. A pregnancy-safe antacid can be suggested by your doctor.

How to Prevent Heartburn

There are steps you can take to prevent heartburn without harming your baby.

Dietary changes

- Instead of three big meals, spread your meals out throughout the day.

- Eat slowly.

- Don't drink with your meals, but between them.

- Steer clear of fried, hot, or greasy foods.

- Don't consume citrus fruits or juice.

Other tips

- Sit up straight while eating.

- Avoid eating after midnight.

- Don't lie down immediately after a meal.

- Keep the foot of your bed lower than the head of your bed, or put pillows under your shoulders.

Stretch Marks

Stretch marks are a normal side effect of your skin expanding to accommodate the growing baby and uterus. Depending on your skin color, they can either be red, purple, pink, or brown. They can develop on your breasts, tummy, arms, hips, thighs, and buttocks.

Not everyone gets them, but if they do appear during pregnancy, they eventually fade... but never really go away. If you get them, blame genetics and your mom.

On the upside, they serve as a constant reminder of your adorable child and a stamp of pride for all the labor that goes with being pregnant!

There isn't anything in particular that you can do to prevent them. Topical or exterior treatments aren't effective since they form deep within your skin, primarily in connective tissues. It's also largely out of your hands because hormones and heredity play a role.

There are some things you can do to lower the likelihood of developing stretch marks and/or lessen their visual impact. It's important to start these precautions before your tummy starts to grow and continue them throughout your pregnancy:

- Apply cream or lotion to your skin every day to keep it hydrated. Even if you don't see stretch marks, do it anyway; it helps with itching too.

- Drinking plenty of water will help you stay hydrated and keep your skin smooth and less susceptible to stretch marks.

- Avoid coffee when pregnant, as it may increase the likelihood of getting stretch marks.

- Maintain a nutritious and healthy diet. Skin health can be supported by a balanced diet high in protein, zinc, and vitamins A, C, and D.

To many, stretch marks are natural and beautiful, but we have to acknowledge that there are people who just don't like the look of them and want to be able to lessen their appearance. Here are some treatments that may minimize their appearance:

- **Creams**: The easiest and most cost-effective solution. Some creams contain ingredients like tretinoin and other retinoids, which are derived from vitamin A. These assist with collagen production on the skin's surface.

- **Light and laser therapy**: Similar to cream, light, and laser therapy can increase elasticity and stimulate the creation of collagen.

- **Hyaluronic acid, micro-needling, and microdermabrasion**: These are more invasive procedures that can also stimulate collagen production. Additionally, they minimize the appearance of stretch marks by helping them integrate with the surrounding skin. Applying hyaluronic acid to the skin everyday can also treat stretch marks.

Like with most medical procedures, talk to your doctor before attempting any of these.

Second Trimester Visits

Every time you see your doctor, they'll check your vitals (weight and blood pressure). Use your visits as a chance to express any concerns you might have. Besides looking out for your well-being, every visit is special because it's a chance for you to see the baby move and hear their heartbeat. Ideally, these moments should be shared with both parents, but it's not always possible. If the father has to miss out for some reason, invite a friend, your mom, or your sister to share in the celebration because every time you see your baby on the screen or hear their heartbeat, that is what it feels like.

With regards to the baby, your doctor will:

- **Assess fetal movement**: Try and take note of how much your baby's moving as soon as you start to feel flutters or kicks, and let your doctor know.

- **Listen to baby's heartbeat**: A Doppler device may be used to detect your baby's heartbeat. It perceives motion and then conveys it as sound.

- **Track baby's growth**: Size can be determined by measuring the distance between the pubic bone and the top of your uterus. This is called "fundal height." This measurement is in centimeters, and usually corresponds with the number of weeks you've been pregnant, give or take 2 cm, after 20 weeks of pregnancy.

Other tests you can look forward to:

- **Genetic tests**: These tests are conducted to check for chromosomal or genetic disorders like Down syndrome or spina bifida. Should your results be a cause for concern, your doctor will suggest an amniocentesis.

- **Fetal ultrasounds**: Imaging that allows you to see images of a developing baby inside the womb using high-frequency sound waves. A thorough ultrasound can assist your doctor in assessing the fetal anatomy, and give you a chance to learn the baby's gender.

- **Blood tests**: Between weeks 24 and 28, you might get tested to ascertain your blood count, iron levels, and to check for gestational diabetes. You may also need a test to look for Rh-antibodies if you've got Rh-negative blood. It's a genetic condition that refers to a particular protein located on the surface of red blood cells. If your baby's blood is Rh-positive and it mixes with yours, antibodies can form. Without treatment, the antibodies can cross the placenta and destroy the developing baby's red blood cells.

You're getting to a stage in your pregnancy where you're almost *settled in*. You've had a couple of doctor's visits, you're feeling a little better, and this is around the time you'll potentially start to show. It's time to start thinking about how and when to let people know.

Making the Announcement: When Is the Best Time?

Pregnancy has many milestones, but a really important one is sharing the news with friends and family. There's always the possibility that you could run into problems early on in the pregnancy, so choosing when to share the news is a delicate thing. Different moms are ultimately going to decide what's best for them and when to share, but there are a few things to consider.

A lot of couples prefer to postpone the announcement until after the first trimester. This is because miscarriages generally occur in the first 12 weeks.

There are some mothers, however, who choose to share the news early because they've had miscarriages before and prefer to have the support of friends and family should it happen again.

These are some of the milestones you should hit before announcing:

- First ultrasound

- Baby bump development

- First anatomy scan

You should feel supported regardless of when you decide to announce your pregnancy. Whether you're expecting your first or fourth child, being pregnant can be a difficult journey. Always discuss any worries you have with your doctor, who may then direct you to a local support group where you can meet other expectant moms in person.

Worker Rights: Should I Tell My Boss?

Women make up 50% of the labor market, and 85% of them will have children throughout their working years. Despite this, finding the ideal time and way to let your employer know you're expecting is daunting. It can get pretty convoluted because letting them know right away seems like the professional thing to do, but doing that might end with you being passed up for opportunities. Your professional growth and the likelihood of receiving raises and promotions may be impacted by your sharing as well.

What Are My Rights and the Legal Requirements for Notice?

When to reveal your pregnancy is not subject to any legal requirements. All you need to do is ask for leave at least 30 days before your planned delivery date if your firm is covered by the Family and Medical Leave Act.

That said, it would be wiser to disclose earlier because women who conceal their pregnancies for extended periods have been found to experience more anxiety while engaging with coworkers than their counterparts who are upfront about it.

I'd suggest letting your employer know towards the end of the first trimester, because your chances of miscarriage are lower, and you may start showing at this time. This way, there'll be enough time to discuss your absence and develop a suitable transition plan for your replacement. There are times when it's necessary to reveal your pregnancy sooner, like if you get sick often and need to schedule doctor visits more frequently.

Also, you have legal protection against discrimination: Pregnancy-based discrimination is illegal under the Pregnancy Discrimination Act (PDA). It prohibits it in all areas of work, including hiring, firing, salary, job assignments, promotions, layoffs, training, and fringe benefits like leave and health insurance.

Even though the law protects us, discrimination still happens. In the last ten years, more than 50,000 accusations of pregnancy discrimination have been leveled against employers.

If you believe you're being victimized, there are steps you can take, like reporting any incidents to the Equal Employment Opportunity Commission and Fair Employment Practices Agencies.

With work sorted, there are things at home that need tending to.

Your Sex Life in Trimesters Two and Three

Some couples believe that sexual activity during pregnancy raises the possibility of miscarriage. But, unless your doctor or midwife has specifically advised against it, it's completely safe.

Sex in the Second Trimester

Throughout the second trimester, women's sexual preferences and habits change. Couples may discover that they revive their sex life at this point in the pregnancy because the expectant mom might be embracing the changes in her body. This could lead to an increase in libido.

But for a lot of couples, it's the opposite. They experience what's called a "five-month crisis." This might happen because some women tend to withdraw into themselves, which makes their partners feel isolated.

Some couples opt to abstain when pregnant because they don't feel comfortable. Despite not engaging in direct sexual activity, they employ various strategies to feel sexually satisfied in their relationship.

Sex in the Third Trimester

Even in the third trimester, your partner will still be very interested in sex, but naturally, there will be a decline in activity because of discomfort. Many women in their third trimester worry that orgasms will cause their uteri to contract. Some also start to feel less attractive, become less willing to engage, and then start to feel anxious about their partners' sexual gratification.

A good compromise for a lot of couples is rear or side entry positions as opposed to the ones that need anybody to be on top.

Potential Risks and When to Avoid Sex in Pregnancy

Sexual activity may increase your chance of developing an infection or bleeding before giving birth if you have a placenta praevia.

Penetrative sex should be avoided while pregnant if:

- You have placenta previa.

- You're bleeding heavily.

- Your waters' broken.

- You have cervical issues.

- You're having multiples or are very late in your pregnancy.

Should you or your partner be engaging in sexual activity outside of the relationship, always use condoms to prevent yourself or your unborn child from contracting any STDs.

Depression During Pregnancy

We've all heard about postpartum depression, but have you heard about antenatal depression?

We go through so many emotions while we're pregnant. Most are positive, but according to research, roughly 7% of pregnant women experience depression (Mayo Clinic, 2019).

Depression is the most common mental illness, and it affects women more than it does men, especially during our reproductive years.

Sometimes It Goes Unnoticed

The symptoms of depression can be mistaken for normal pregnancy symptoms because they're so similar. Low energy levels, increased sleeping time, and changes in appetite. It's very easy for your doctor to miss.

We're in the 21st century, but there's still a stigma attached to depression, so some women may be hesitant to discuss changes in their mood during pregnancy with their doctors. Also, there is a propensity to prioritize a woman's physical health during pregnancy over her mental health.

Risk Factors
- Anxiety
- Stress
- Prior depression
- Inadequate emotional support
- Unplanned pregnancy
- Intimate partner violence

Signs and Symptoms
- Extreme anxiety regarding your baby

- Low self-esteem, and feeling like you won't be a good parent

- Not enjoying activities you once did

- Being unresponsive to reassurance

- Not complying with prenatal care

- Using drugs

- Poor weight gain due to insufficient diet

- Suicidal thoughts

Treatment Options

Untreated depression may lead to you not being receptive to prenatal care, eating the nutritious meals your baby needs, or having the motivation to take care of yourself. Moreover, you are more likely to have postpartum depression and trouble bonding with your child in the future.

Your options are psychotherapy or medication like antidepressants; this all depends on the severity of your depression.

Your Baby's Development

TOMATO

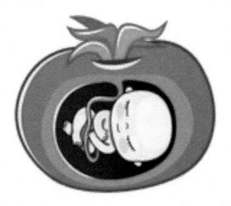

This is the start of the *honeymoon period*. Your uterus is expanding very quickly, roughly at the same rate as your baby, and it's moving higher up into your abdominal cavity, so you may start to notice your belly becoming a little pudge.

In contrast to trimester one, you are probably feeling more energized and somewhat "normal." It's around this time that you'll be a lot more peckish, and eating more means more gas, indigestion, and bloating.

Baby is around 4–5 inches in length and weighs around three ounces. Roughly the size of a tomato. They're also starting to gain a bit of muscle mass and back muscles, so their body will start to straighten out more and look less bean-like.

Due to the increase in muscles, they can actually make facial expressions. Baby's eyes are no longer on the sides of their heads, and they have eyelashes and brows.

Baby's heart is working really hard, pumping about 25 quarts of blood everyday.

Chapter 5: Month Five

Fetal Movements

Monitoring your unborn child's movement is an excellent idea, especially during the third trimester. This way, you can alert your doctor for further investigation if you feel a decrease in movement.

When Does It Start?

Some people refer to those initial, fluttery sensations as "quickening." You might feel something initially, and then question whether you actually did, because those early movements may feel like bubbles or like a gentle flutter. Some people even mistake them for gas.

You will start feeling movement in your second trimester. It can start anywhere between 16 and 22 weeks, but if it's your first pregnancy, it can happen later on—possibly between 20 and 22 weeks. If you've been pregnant before, you might be more aware of them a little earlier, possibly at the 16-week mark. Every pregnancy is different, though, and there's no specific time to feel movement.

What's It Like in the Second Trimester?

During the second trimester, your baby's movements can be a little erratic. It will start off with the flutters, and then the actual fetal movements will start to happen a little more regularly and intensely because the baby's warming up for the Olympics. Eventually, you may start to feel some stretches and possibly even some punches and kicks as your baby grows, and its movements become more intense.

What's It Like in the Third Trimester?

You might begin to recognize certain patterns in your baby's movements at some point during this final trimester. Maybe there are specific hours of the day or night when he/she is more active.

The movements will become bigger and more forceful, and occasionally you might feel a particularly ferocious kick or punch. If your baby is moving beneath your skin, you might be able to see it.

Unfortunately, by this time, your baby is beginning to run out of room to move about. But that just means they're becoming stronger, gaining weight, and gaining some of that healthy baby fat. Since the baby can't stretch and move around as freely, they may start to move less, but you should still feel some sort of movement. If you become worried, your doctor might suggest a kick count.

Kick Count

You choose a time of day and count how many times your baby kicks or moves throughout that period. It's also called a "fetal movement count" (FMC). There are apps you can download to keep track of things.

For the most accurate comparison, it's best to perform a kick count at the same time every day. Keep an eye on the baby's movement and time how long it takes to get to ten kicks.

Try having a snack, shifting positions, and then continuing your count for another hour if your baby doesn't kick, wriggle, or poke you ten times in that period. You can stop the count if you get to 10 before the second hour is up.

So if you keep track of your baby's kicks and notice a day when they stop, tell your doctor as soon as you can.

What Causes a Decrease in Movement?

There are many reasons why your baby's movements might slow down. Most of them aren't alarming, but sometimes not feeling your baby kick could be an indication that something's wrong. If you see a dramatic decrease in activity over several hours, you should call your doctor.

Benign causes:

- Your baby is too little for you to feel anything. This is normal early on in the second trimester.

- You engaged in sexual activity. After intercourse, some babies become more active and others become less active. Your baby may fall asleep if you reach orgasm or because of the sexual motions. It can go either way in both the second and third trimesters.

- You've been physically active. If you move around a lot, your baby may fall asleep, or you might be too busy moving around to notice anything that's going on with the baby.

- Your baby has dozed off. Babies normally sleep for 20- to 45-minute intervals all throughout the day. They can spend up to 95% of their time asleep by 38 weeks of gestation.

- Your baby's too big to be mobile. As your due date draws near, your baby is approaching their birth weight and size.

- Your baby's preparing for birth. They may be less active if their head has sunk into the pelvis in preparation for delivery.

How to Increase Movement

If you're feeling uneasy and want to encourage your baby to say hello, here are some things you can do to get them moving:

- Move around.

- Have a snack or a sugary beverage, like orange juice.

- Speak to your baby.

- Light up your tummy with a flashlight.

- Try to feel your baby in your belly by pushing or poking at it gently.

Once your baby starts kicking, you'll probably start to look forward to it, and it'll be the highlight of most of your days. On the other hand, the kicking might keep you awake at times.

Trouble Sleeping?

Sleep can be so elusive during pregnancy. You start off sleeping all the time and end up hardly getting any at all. Many sleep issues are caused by physical discomfort, hormonal changes, excitement, and worry related to becoming a new mother. In fact, it's estimated that at least half of pregnant women have trouble sleeping.

Sleep is a really important part of prenatal care, but it escapes many of us. Let's delve into sleeping issues, the best sleeping positions, and some tips on how to maximize your sleep during pregnancy.

Common Sleep Disorders and Problems During Pregnancy

- **Obstructive sleep apnea**

  Many women start to snore once they fall pregnant because of weight gain and nasal congestion. Should you experience snoring, gasping, and periodic breathing pauses that impair sleep quality, you've developed obstructive sleep apnea. It can obstruct the flow of oxygen to your fetus and raise the risk of preeclampsia, gestational diabetes, and C-sections. It is estimated that one in five pregnant women experiences this, so consult your doctor if you notice any signs.

- **Gastroesophageal reflux disorder**

  GERD for short. It's like ongoing acid reflux, and it can really affect your sleep across all trimesters. It affects about half of pregnant women in the third trimester and a quarter in the first. If left untreated, it can damage the esophagus.

- **Restless leg syndrome**

  People with RLS have uncontrollable urges to move their legs due to sensations that are best described as crawling, tickling, or itching. The symptoms tend to be more severe when one is at rest, and that makes it difficult to fall asleep. Up to a third of pregnant women may get RLS during the third trimester.

Why Is Sleep Such a Big Deal?

Getting quality sleep is crucial for both mom and baby. Sleepless nights eventually result in exhaustion and daytime sleepiness. Sleep aids memory, learning, appetite, mood, and decision-making—all of which are imperatives while getting ready to welcome a newborn home.

Your immune system suffers when you're deprived of quality sleep on a regular basis. It's why sleep has such a profound effect on maternal and fetal health. Sleep also helps manage your blood sugar, so if you're not getting enough, you run the risk of developing gestational diabetes.

Women with unbalanced sleeping patterns in early pregnancy are prone to developing high blood pressure in their third trimester. This can lead to preeclampsia, which in turn raises your risk of preterm delivery and long-term complications for the kidneys, heart, and other organs.

There is new evidence that poor sleep during pregnancy is a precursor to babies with sleep problems who cry incessantly.

Treatment for Pregnancy-Related Sleep Issues

There are several methods for reducing sleep issues without needing medication. The key to having better sleep is controlling pregnancy-related sleep disturbances and practicing good sleep hygiene. Try some of these methods before opting for medication.

Best Sleeping Positions

The ideal position is on your left side with your legs slightly curled. This way, your baby's oxygen and nutrients are distributed niccly, and there's more blood flow to the uterus, heart, and kidneys. The right side is okay too; it's just not as ideal.

If you're not used to sleeping on your side, you can use a couple of extra pillows to help you feel comfortable. If you'd like to ease pressure on your lower back, put a lightweight pillow between your knees or tuck a wedge pillow under your tummy for support. Body pillows are also really good and less complicated to navigate.

Sleeping on your back can give you back pain and put a strain on your vena cava as the uterus expands. It's one of your main veins, so if it's obstructed, you could start to feel lightheaded.

You're not expected to avoid sleeping on your back altogether; you can do it in short bouts. Just try your best to avoid it as much as humanly possible.

Once your belly grows past a certain point, it will be impossible to sleep on your tummy.

Sleep Hygiene

The following practices may help minimize insomnia and enhance overall sleep quality:

- Maintain a calm, quiet, dark bedroom, and only use the bed for sleeping and sexual activity.

- Make sleep a priority, maintain a regular bedtime, and plan naps earlier in the day to avoid disturbing your nocturnal sleep.

- Prepare your body for sleep by reading a book, taking a bath, or engaging in another activity you find peaceful.

- Consider getting a nightlight to make those nighttime bathroom breaks easier to navigate.

- To lower your risk of GERD, stay away from coffee, spicy foods, and big meals too close to bedtime.

- Turn off all screens at least an hour before bedtime and avoid bringing electronics into the bedroom.

- Workout regularly, and try to do so earlier in the day.

- While it's important to stay hydrated throughout the day, cutting back on liquids a couple of hours before bed will help you avoid nighttime trips to the bathroom.

- If you have trouble falling asleep, get up and do something else until you're tired.

- If you're feeling stressed, seek help from your partner, friends, or doctor. You may also find it helpful to get a journal you can jot your thoughts down in before bed.

Oral Health Conditions During Pregnancy

- Hormonal changes that intensify the body's response to microorganisms in the gum tissue can cause gingivitis.

- Cavities can develop as a result of dietary changes, like increased snacking, which increases mouth acidity. They can also come from vomiting, dry mouth, or poor oral hygiene brought on by nausea and vomiting.

- Pyogenic granuloma, or granuloma gravidarum, is a spherical growth that typically has a thin cord of tissue connecting it to the gingiva. It may form as a result of hormonal changes.

- Due to all the vomiting, erosion could occur. Avoid brushing the teeth immediately after vomiting, because the teeth can become exposed to stomach acids. To neutralize the acid, rinse with a water and baking soda solution. You can make it with 1 cup of water and a spoonful of baking soda.

Good daily oral hygiene is so important because you're at an increased risk of getting gingivitis and developing cavities. Brush twice daily with a soft-bristle toothbrush and fluoride toothpaste. Flossing would be helpful too.

High Blood Pressure and Preeclampsia

Gestational hypertension develops when a woman experiences high blood pressure during pregnancy without any other cardiac or kidney issues, or protein in the urine. It's usually discovered after 20 weeks of pregnancy or just before delivery. It normally subsides once you give birth, but some women are more likely to develop chronic hypertension.

Preeclampsia is basically gestational hypertension paired with proteinuria. Proteinuria is the presence of protein in the urine, which can be a sign that there is some kidney damage and, in some cases, multiple organ damage.

In the US, preeclampsia affects roughly one in every 25 pregnancies. Once a woman starts experiencing seizures, her condition worsens, and she develops eclampsia, which is a medical emergency.

Symptoms include:

- Difficulty breathing

- Unusual weight gain

- Nausea and vomiting

- Pain in the upper stomach

- Face and hand swelling

- Cloudy vision, seeing spots, or experiencing changes in eyesight

- Persistent headaches

Preeclampsia can set in after birth. It's called "postpartum preeclampsia." The symptoms are the same, and it can happen to women who didn't experience preeclampsia while pregnant. Your healthcare team can usually tell if it's happening a couple of days after birth, but sometimes it can take up to six weeks to manifest.

If you experience symptoms, call 911 right away or inform your healthcare professional. You might need immediate medical attention.

Gestational Diabetes

Gestational diabetes is diagnosed during pregnancy. It's the same as other forms of diabetes in the sense that it affects your blood sugar. Elevated blood sugar can be harmful to you and your baby.

You can manage it by eating well, working out, and taking medication if necessary. If you have it during pregnancy, your blood sugar should go back to normal very soon after delivery. You would, however, be at risk of developing type 2 diabetes and have to undergo testing more often.

Gestational diabetes has no apparent indications or symptoms apart from increased thirst and more frequent urination. You will most likely find out through testing, as that's part of your prenatal care.

Causes

It's still unknown why some women develop gestational diabetes and others don't. Weight gain is usually the main suspect, though.

Normally, your hormones control your blood sugar levels. So when you're pregnant and your hormones are out of whack, your body has a tougher time effectively processing the sugar in your blood. This causes a spike in your blood glucose levels.

Risk Factors

- Overweight/obesity

- Not engaging in physical activity

- Being pre-diabetic

- Having Polycystic Ovary Syndrome (POCS)

- Having immediate family with diabetes

- Having delivered a baby over 9 lbs in the past

- Ethnicity. Namely: Asian American, American Indian, African American, Hispanic

Complications

- **Breathing difficulties**: Early babies may develop respiratory distress syndrome, which makes breathing extremely hard for them.

- **C-section**: Uncontrolled diabetes increases a woman's likelihood of needing a C-section to deliver the baby.

- **High birth weight**: Your baby may become too big if your blood sugar levels are above the recommended range. Babies who weigh 9 pounds or more are more likely to experience delivery injuries, become trapped in the birth canal, or require a C-section.

- **Hypoglycemia**: Some babies born to moms with GD can suffer hypoglycemia just after birth. Their low blood sugar may lead to them experiencing seizures. The baby's blood sugar level can be brought back to normal by early feedings and, occasionally, an intravenous glucose solution.

- **Obesity and type 2 diabetes**: Babies born to moms with GD may experience obesity or type 2 diabetes later in life.

- **Preterm birth**: Moms with diabetes are more likely to experience preterm labor, especially if the baby is already very big.

- **Stillbirth**: If left untreated, gestational diabetes can lead to the baby's passing away either before birth or soon after.

Prevention

- Eat nutritious food

- Be physically active

- Start your pregnancy off at a healthy weight

- Avoid gaining more weight than is advised

- Attend all antenatal checkups

Anemia

When you're iron deficient, your red blood cells aren't healthy enough to carry enough oxygen to your body's tissues. Your body needs more iron when you are pregnant because of the increased blood volume. If your iron levels are insufficient and you don't supplement, you could develop anemia.

Risk Factors

- Having two consecutive pregnancies

- Expecting multiples

- Frequent vomiting

- Having insufficient iron in your diet
- Heavy menstrual flow before pregnancy
- A history of anemia

Symptoms

- Headache
- Pale skin
- Difficulty breathing
- Craving ice (PICA)
- Dizziness
- Weakness
- Fatigue

Symptoms of severe anemia:

- Low blood pressure
- Rapid heartbeat
- Trouble concentrating

Treatment and Prevention

Iron is usually present in prenatal vitamins, but in some instances, your medical practitioner may advise you to take an additional iron supplement. You need at least 27 milligrams of iron per day while you're pregnant.

Maintaining a healthy diet that includes iron-rich foods helps a lot. You can get iron from fish, poultry, or lean red meat. You can also get it from breakfast cereals, leafy green veggies, peas, or dried beans.

Your body absorbs iron from meat and other animal products a lot easier. So if you're a vegetarian or if you're opting to get your iron from non-animal products, combine them with other elements high in vitamin C. You can use juices like tomato and orange or have some strawberries on the side. Refrain from drinking fruit juices that have been fortified with calcium because they make it harder to absorb iron.

Skin Discoloration

Most of the changes that happen to your skin are harmless, but some could irritate you and cause you discomfort. Here are some changes you can anticipate and some advice on when to consult your midwife or doctor:

- changes in skin tone (pigmentation), like darkening of the neck, inner thighs, breasts, nipples, and parts of the face

- moles, freckles, and birthmarks becoming more pigmented

- blemishes or acne

- varicose veins

- spider veins

- skin tags

- crimson or darkened palms

- skin sensitivity

- itchy skin

Pregnancy-related skin changes are harmless to both you and your unborn child.

Skin issues might occasionally be an indication of an underlying condition that a doctor should examine. Keep in mind that these illnesses are quite rare:

- **Intrahepatic cholestasis**

Almost everybody itches during pregnancy, but a small percentage of women struggle with severe itching due to a liver condition called "intrahepatic cholestasis." Your body begins to accumulate bile acids as a result of the illness.

There's no visible rash, and you might notice that the itching is more pronounced on the soles of your feet and palms of your hands. It's usually worse at night. Thankfully, things tend to improve shortly after delivery.

See your doctor or midwife if you are experiencing these symptoms so they can order some blood tests to determine how well your liver is functioning.

To stop the itching, your doctor may recommend lotions or medications.

- **Pemphigoid gestationis**

A rare illness that causes an itchy rash that turns into blisters during pregnancy.

This occurs when your body mounts an immunological reaction, which may be brought on by tiny amounts of placental material getting into your bloodstream. It usually happens in the second and third trimesters.

It's crucial to see your doctor or midwife if you get an itchy rash, because the itching can be lessened, and sore regions soothed with lotions and ointments they prescribe.

If you observe any changes in the color, size, form, or thickness of a mole or birthmark, always talk to a doctor.

Why Does Your Skin Get Darker?

Your skin will get darker during pregnancy. It might be all over, or it might be in little patches. You may also observe the following:

- Dark patches on your face (pigmentation). This is referred to as melasma or the pregnant mask. Hormonal changes that occur may cause melasma by temporarily increasing the amount of melanin your body generates. It is estimated that this happens to up to 75% of expectant mothers (*Melasma: Treatment, Causes & Prevention*, 2020).

- Your neck, inner thighs, genitalia, and areolas turn darker.

- Your birthmarks, moles, freckles, and recent scars start to darken.

- The region surrounding your belly button, as well as your armpits and inner thighs, may darken if you have brown or black skin. After birth, these areas will gradually become lighter again, but some may remain a little darker than before.

Your patches might become darker in the sun, making them more visible. Wear a wide-brimmed hat outside, use sunscreen with an SPF of 50 or higher, and try to stay as much as you can in the shade to protect your skin.

It's normal to feel self-conscious about your patches, but they will probably go away within a year of the birth of your child. Concealer, foundation, and tinted moisturizer can all help even out your skin tone in the interim.

After the birth of their children, one in ten mothers discovers that their black spots persist. If this is the case, your doctor may suggest some treatment options.

What is the Dark Line Running Up Your Bump?

Linea nigra is the scientific term for the vertical line that runs down the center of your belly. Normally, it extends from the top of your pubic bone to the center of your belly, but it can occasionally cross over to end just below your breastbone.

It starts to show in the second trimester, and it's a normal aspect of pregnancy. But if you don't get one, it's not a cause for concern.

It's located on the abdominal muscles, so it expands and widens as your baby grows, but it's just due to hormone-related pigmentation.

Once you give birth, it starts to disappear and should be gone within a few months.

Does Pregnancy Glow Exist?

There are some upsides to all the changes happening in your body, you get a luminous, slightly flushed glow that makes you look so good during pregnancy. It's due to fluctuating hormone levels, increased sebum (oil) production, and increased blood flow throughout your body.

The only drawback is that when your body retains moisture, your legs and ankles may swell. Also, if you have any spots on your face, neck, or chest, the blood flow to your skin may make them more obvious. Like most things, a few months after giving birth, these things will stop happening.

Drinking plenty of water can really aid your body in eliminating extra water. Maintaining good hydration will also be amazing for your skin.

Why Are My Veins More Pronounced on My Cheek?

- Acne: It results in broken blood vessels, often known as "spider veins." When they are swollen or dilated just beneath the surface of your skin, you get tiny, red lines that spread out into the shape of a web.

- Rosacea: This condition results in swollen veins that cause the skin to flush and turn red. Spider veins are usually present in people with rosacea.

How Can I Look After My Skin?

- Avoid over-cleansing because this can make your skin dry. Use a fragrance-free makeup remover or gentle soap to wash your face twice daily. This will be plenty to keep your skin clear and young-looking.

- Go for pore-clearing water-based solutions rather than oil-based ones. Search for products with the designations "noncomedogenic" or "pH-balanced."

- Avoid picking or squeezing your pimples to prevent scarring on your skin

- Use acne creams and treatments only on your doctor's recommendation. Certain acne remedies should not be used during pregnancy because they could harm the developing fetus.

- Keep up a balanced diet.

Your Baby's Development

MANGOSTEEN

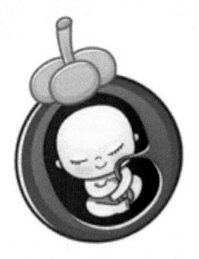

You are officially halfway through your pregnancy at 20 weeks along! Take a deep breath if you're not too congested to do so. Your hormones are working in your favor this month, as they're triggering an uptick in circulation. This means your nails will grow faster, and your hair will be thicker and longer.

Baby measures 6.5 inches long and weighs about 10 ounces, like a mangosteen. If you haven't already found out the baby's gender, now would be as good a time as any.

If you're carrying a boy, his testicles have developed in his abdomen this month and will begin to descend into the scrotum. If you're carrying a girl, her genitals may not be as clear on an ultrasound, but they're there, and her vaginal canal is slowly developing. She's got a fully formed uterus and ovaries with millions of eggs inside.

This is a really nice time for baby in the pregnancy because there's still lots of space to move around. Speaking of kicking, if you haven't felt any yet, it should start soon.

Chapter 6: Month Six

This is quite a good month for most women. You're relatively far along in the pregnancy, but you're not experiencing extreme discomfort like you would in trimester three. Your baby bump is probably nice and round now, and you may love the look of your cute belly.

Something that couples enjoy doing is having a babymoon— one last holiday to connect as a couple before the baby comes. It takes a bit of extra planning, though, because you're carrying precious cargo.

Is It Safe to Travel By Air?

A lot of women travel while pregnant, but it's still important to consider any issues that can arise when traveling abroad. Moreover, consider how you would access high-quality medical care in the nations you are visiting. Instead of waiting to get the necessary vaccinations while pregnant, get them all before.

According to the American College of Obstetricians and Gynecologists, the safest time to travel is in the second trimester—between 14 and 28 weeks—because it's when you feel your best. Moreover, your chance of spontaneous abortion and early labor is at its lowest. It's advised that you stay within a 300-mile radius of your home during the third trimester, or from 25 to 40 weeks. This is due to issues like phlebitis, elevated blood pressure, and false or preterm labor. For domestic flights, women are often prohibited from flying after 36 weeks, and for international flights, after 28 to 35 weeks. But the final decision should be between you and your doctor or midwife.

There are a few conditions under which you are likely to be prohibited from flying to countries with pre-travel vaccines:

- Incompetent cervix

- Pregnant with multiples

- History of early labor or early membrane rupture

- Cardiomyopathy or congestive heart failure

- Severe anemia

- History of blood clots

- Gereatric pregnancy

- Prior reproductive issues or difficulties getting pregnant

- History of toxemia, hypertension, or diabetes during any pregnancy

- Past or present placental anomalies

- History of ectopic pregnancy or miscarriage

- Threatened miscarriage or vaginal bleeding

Tips for Traveling While Pregnant

- Prior to your trip, try to prepare for any problems or emergencies that might arise. Verify that your health insurance is still in effect while you're traveling. In the event that you give birth while away, make sure the plan will cover your child as well. Consider getting supplementary travel and medical evacuation insurance.

- Look into the local hospitals before you go. Women who are in their third trimester of pregnancy should seek out facilities that can handle cesarean sections, toxemia, and other pregnancy-related problems.

- Make arrangements for prenatal care in advance if you'll need it while traveling.

- Know your blood type and confirm the places you'll be visiting to screen blood for hepatitis B and HIV.

- Verify that safe foods and drinks like pasteurized milk and bottled water are available where you're going.

- When traveling by air, request an aisle seat at the bulkhead. That way, you'll have more space and comfort. If you experience morning sickness, make travel arrangements for a time of day when you typically feel good.

- On a calm flight, try to move your legs every 30 minutes. Avoid blood clots by frequently flexing and extending your ankles (thrombophlebitis).

- To stay hydrated, consume lots of liquids because the humidity in aircraft cabins is minimal.

As amazing as month six is, it's not without its discomforts. These are some things you may start to experience:

Hemorrhoids

These are inflamed veins around your anus that can make going to the bathroom a very painful experience. They typically go away once you give birth.

When hemorrhoids are external, they're on the anus, and when they're internal, they're in your rectum. Your rectum is the portion of your large intestine that connects to your anus. They are an uncomfortable but typical aspect of pregnancy, but the good news is that they're relatively easy to cure at home.

Symptoms

You can actually have hemorrhoids and not exhibit any symptoms, but the most common ones are:

- Discomfort while passing a stool.

- Your anus and its surrounding area itch.

- An internal hemorrhoid that causes excruciating pain outside of your anus (prolapsed hemorrhoid).

- Blood in your stool, on the toilet, or on the toilet paper you used after relieving yourself (usually from an internal hemorrhoid).

*Treatment **Options***

Relieve constipation: Regular bowel movements might relieve some of the pressure on your hemorrhoids. The less time you spend straining yourself, the less pressure you apply to these veins. You can:

- Drink 8–12 cups of water per day.

- Eat up to 30 grams of fiber everyday.

- Take a pregnancy-safe laxative.

Use home remedies:

- To relieve mild pain or discomfort, apply pure aloe vera or food-grade coconut oil.

- To relieve the itch and pain, apply witch hazel.

- To relieve itching, apply dry or wet baking soda directly onto your hemorrhoids.

- Sit in a tub with 2 to 3 inches of warm water, or take a sitz bath. The tense muscles surrounding your anus will start to relax, and your blood flow may be improved in the water.

Medication: If constipation is the main problem, ask your doctor to recommend a laxative, hemorrhoid cream or fiber supplement. It's better to consult with your doctor on this before opting for any over-the-counter medication. Your doctor or midwife is your best bet at ensuring that you get solutions that are both safe and effective.

Failing these, your doctor might be able to recommend a procedure to remove them that's safe for both you and your baby.

What Are Anal Fissures?

Same ballpark, just a little different. Anal fissures are tears in the anus.

Hemorrhoids and fissures share similar symptoms and can both be uncomfortable and painful. They can also result in bleeding, which you'll see either in your stool or on the toilet paper you use after wiping. The bleeding is harmless, but if you're really worried, don't hesitate to call your doctor. They'll be able to confirm the source of your bleeding and whether or not it's from a more serious condition.

Belly Button Protrusion

We don't usually give our navels much thought, but once we fall pregnant, our belly buttons are one of the many changes we'll see on our bodies.

You're likely to notice the change in your second trimester. Your abdomen moves forward as your uterus continues to grow, and then your belly button eventually protrudes because of your expanding abdomen.

It's completely harmless, but some women have noted that clothing rubbing against it irritates it. If it bothers you, you can wear a belly button cover or a support tool like a tummy sleeve.

Some ladies do experience pain, but there's no universally accepted medical explanation for why some women do. Some people think it has to do with the belly button's location at the thinnest part of the abdominal wall.

Like a lot of things, it usually goes back to normal a couple of months after you've given birth.

What's an Umbilical Hernia?

Sometimes your protruding belly button can actually be an umbilical hernia. It happens when a small hole in your abdominal wall allows abdominal tissue, like the small intestine, to protrude. It can be very uncomfortable.

Symptoms

- A soft lump near your navel that is more pronounced when you are laying down.

- A nagging pain near your navel.

- Some discomfort when you cough, sneeze, or lean over.

Causes

Most umbilical hernias are congenital. They just go unnoticed until your abdomen starts stretching,

Treatment

It's best to leave it alone if it's not causing discomfort. Some ladies rub the lump until the bulge goes inward, and to prevent them from expanding even more, some ladies use belly bands.

After your pregnancy, the hernia will probably start to heal. Your doctor might suggest certain exercises you can do to help it along.

Surgery may be advised by your doctor in some circumstances, but it won't be done until after you've given birth.

Stillbirth

The untimely loss of a pregnancy in any trimester is heartbreaking. Miscarriages usually occur within the first three months, but they can occasionally happen after 20 weeks. Those cases are referred to as stillbirths.

Even though you might never know what led to your loss, it's important to understand that it's highly unlikely that anything you did or didn't do contributed to it. Most miscarriages are the result of issues with the baby's development.

Other causes include:

- **Chromosome or genetic abnormalities**: these occur by chance, but sometimes they're passed down by parents. You can request blood tests to check your chromosomes and assess the likelihood of the same issue arising again.

- **Infection**: some infections affect the baby directly, and others are in the amniotic fluid. Sometimes bacteria from the vagina gets into the womb.

- **Structural abnormalities**: these occur when there's a problem with a baby's development. One example is a congenital heart defect.

- **Problems with the uterus or cervix**: An oddly shaped uterus or a weakened cervix can result in a late loss.

Dealing With Loss

It's normal to experience a great deal of grief and other feelings like guilt, anger, despair, and shock. Those feelings will feel real, but it's never your fault. Everyone reacts differently, so it's important to be honest about your feelings with your spouse and keep in mind that you might not both be processing the loss in the same way. Give yourself time to recover, rely on your loved ones, and think about attending a support group for miscarriage or stillbirth.

Healing

Sometimes you may feel distant, moody, and unable to focus or sleep.

Don't put pressure on yourself to get over your unhappiness. If you can handle your grief as it manifests, your healing will be more thorough. The pain may come back on special occasions like your due date, but with time, things will improve and you'll feel better.

You may be okay physically, but it would help to take a bit of time out. You need time to process, and it may be easier to embrace everything you're going through if you take a break from your usual routine.

Talking

Sharing your story can help you feel less alone and put you on the path to healing. It may seem unpleasant or taboo, but you'll start to see how many people you know have experienced loss and found recovery.

You may find comfort in the most unlikely people, and being transparent about your story, might liberate someone else from the loneliness associated with pregnancy loss and provide them with the strength and confidence to do the same.

If you don't get the response you expected from certain people, bear in mind that people who haven't experienced such a loss can't possibly understand how it feels. Most people actually want to offer comfort but lack the words. If someone says something you deem inappropriate or nothing at all, try not to take it personally.

Support

You won't need to do much Web searching to be reminded that you're not alone. You might find it easier to deal with loss through internet forums. Sometimes it just helps to know you're not the only one going through something.

Ask your ob-gyn or midwife about local pregnancy-loss support groups if you prefer to be face-to-face with people.

Don't give up if you don't enjoy the first one you try; it could take some time to find a group that suits you. Try to learn as much as you can in advance about the group's members to determine whether you'll fit in. (Do they deal more with miscarriages or with stillbirths?)

If a group feels like too much, a counselor might be able to assist you in navigating the feelings you're having and ultimately help you accept your loss.

Your Baby's Development

ARTICHOKE

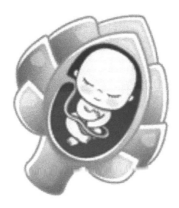

Your belly button may be popping out now, and you could be experiencing round ligament pain. Your ligaments are stretching to support your growing baby.

Baby is measuring in at 11.5 inches and weighs in at around 1.3 pounds. The same as an artichoke. Your baby's bones, muscles, and organs continue to grow and develop. They even have some body fat now.

At this stage, your baby's facial features are starting to take shape. If anything, baby is ready for his/her photo opp. They haven't yet developed pigment. So the baby has white eyebrows, hair, and eyelashes.

Their auditory system develops quickly, so if you play a certain song often enough, they may recognize it and find it calming after birth.

TRIMESTER 3:

Waiting Impatiently

Chapter 7: Month Seven

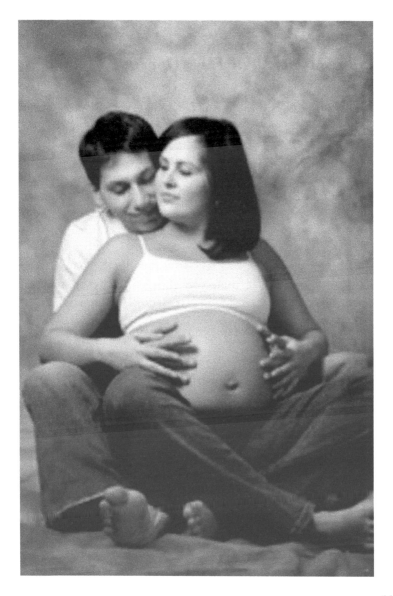

Two months may seem like a long time, but this is the final stretch, and it's getting closer to delivery time. There are things to start thinking about, things to start planning, and things to start implementing.

Birthing Partner: Why Have One?

A birth partner can offer you much-needed support throughout your labor.

You can decide to choose both your partner and a close friend or relative. Just take some time to really consider who you want in the room. If, for any reason, family and friends aren't an option, you can hire a professional like an independent midwife or a doula.

What's important is that you feel at ease with the person you choose. Over and above that, you should have faith in their capacity to keep you at ease and reassured when you are in labor.

Partners

For a lot of dads, witnessing the birth of their child was easily one of their most emotional experiences. But there are some dads who are anxious about being the only support partner.

Likewise, some women worry about their partners' ability to cope, while others don't want them to see them go through labor at all. A good idea is to have two birth partners. That way, they can alternate or take turns looking after you without feeling burned out.

Family and friends

Women have been helping other women give birth since the beginning of time, so it's no wonder a lot of moms-to-be go with female family members in place of their partners. Some women have female family members there in conjunction with their partners.

Your mom is probably the best option because she can let you know what to expect, and since she has firsthand knowledge of the labor process, she can offer you solid support.

Professionals

Independent midwives are a good option if you're planning a homebirth. They can deliver your child and provide you with antenatal and postnatal care. If you choose to deliver at a birthing center, they can support you throughout labor but won't actually deliver the baby.

A doula provides emotional support during labor and delivery. There will be a bit of a rapport because they will get to know you beforehand and will be there to help you emotionally in the days and weeks following the birth of your child. The only thing they can't do is deliver the baby.

Birthing Classes vs. Lamaze

Birthing courses have different philosophies and objectives, but they all offer helpful guidance for labor, delivery, and postpartum issues. Some are focused on how to manage labor pain without drugs. Others start early in a woman's pregnancy and concentrate on the changes that take place for the whole nine months.

Lamaze Technique

Probably the most popular birthing method—it's in all the movies!

Lamaze classes view delivery as a natural and healthy process. They don't encourage or discourage the use of drugs or standard medical procedures during labor and delivery. Instead, they educate expectant mothers about their choices so that they can plan their own labor and delivery. The Lamaze program includes instruction on confidence-building and safe, easy childbirth techniques.

The classes are small, and there are about 12 hours of instruction that provide you with knowledge on:

- A healthy lifestyle

- Assistance during labor

- Breastfeeding

- Breathing exercises for labor

- How to communicate effectively

- Medical procedures

- Pain relief with massage and relaxation techniques

- Positioning yourself in various ways for labor and delivery

- Standard birth, delivery, and early postpartum care

- Using both internal and external focal points to help practice relaxation

Alexander Technique

Your balance, flexibility, coordination, and freedom of movement can all be enhanced by the Alexander Technique. Ideally, you should participate in weekly classes while pregnant, because it's more of an educational process. So, the more you practice, the more you'll gain. Anyone can take these classes, but the objectives for pregnant women include:

- Aid with postpartum healing

- Boost comfort levels during pregnancy

- During delivery, increase the effectiveness of pushing

- Reduce breastfeeding discomfort

HypnoBirthing

Hypnobirthing, also known as the Mongan method, is a laid-back educational approach to natural childbirth. It teaches you self-hypnosis techniques. Instructors place a strong emphasis on prenatal care, parenting, and the consciousness of the unborn child. It's delivered in a series of either four or five classes, each lasting three hours.

The Bradley Method

The Bradley method, also known as husband-coached delivery, gets mom ready to give birth without painkillers and gets dad ready to be mom's birth coach. Although this strategy gets you ready to give birth without drugs, it also gets you ready for unforeseen events like an emergency C-section.

This 12-session program covers:

- Advice for the coach regarding support for the mother

- Breastfeeding

- How to give birth vaginally

- Postpartum care

- Pain management techniques based on relaxation

- The significance of diet and exercise

- Labor rehearsals

If you're unsure about the type of class you want to enroll in, take some time to explore the ones close by, and talk through your options with your doctor. You should also ask where you can find local childbirth classes. Failing that, search online.

Pain Relief in Labor

Labor is hands-down the most painful experience a woman will go through in her lifetime. So learning about all the ways you can ease the pain is so important. Your birth partner/s should also be well informed so they can step in if you need help.

Gas and Air (Entonox) For Labor

It contains both nitrous oxide and oxygen. Although gas and air cannot completely alleviate pain, they can help to lessen it and make it more tolerable. It is simple to use, and you are in complete control.

You hold the mask or mouthpiece while inhaling gas and air through it. You breathe it in just before a contraction starts, since it takes the gas around 15–20 seconds to start working. You should breathe deeply and slowly for the best results.

Side effects:

- There are no adverse effects for you or the child.

- It may cause you to feel dizzy, ill, sleepy, or unable to concentrate, but you can stop using it if this happens.

You might also request an injection of painkillers if gas and air do not sufficiently relieve your discomfort.

Epidural

An epidural is a local anesthesia that numbs the nerves that transmit pain signals from the birth canal to the brain. It doesn't make you feel sick or drowsy. It typically provides total pain relief, so it's really helpful if your labor is protracted and painful.

It can only be administered by an anesthesiologist, so it's not available for home births. Find out if anesthetists are always available at your hospital if you believe you might need one.

Bear in mind that the baby's heart rate must also be remotely (through telemetry) monitored at this time, but many hospitals lack the necessary equipment. Find out from your midwife whether your hospital of choice offers mobile epidurals.

It works most of the time, but it's not always successful. According to the Obstetric Anaesthetists Association, one in ten women who have an epidural during labor end up needing additional painkillers.

Side Effects

- Depending on the local anesthetic used, it may cause your legs to feel heavy.

- It's possible for your blood pressure to drop (hypotension), but it rarely happens because the fluid you get via the drip in your arm aids in maintaining healthy blood pressure.

- The second stage of labor may be prolonged in the event that you're unable to feel your contractions anymore. Your midwife will have to instruct you on when to push, and then she may need the assistance of forceps or a ventouse (instrumental delivery).

- As long as the baby is not displaying any signs of distress, your midwife or doctor will wait longer for the baby's head to drop before you begin pushing. This lowers the likelihood that you'll require an instrumental delivery. They also start weaning you off the anesthesia toward the end of labor, so the effects wear off and you can feel the contractions.

- The epidural may make it difficult for you to urinate. If so, a catheter might be inserted into your bladder to assist you.

- It may cause a headache. But that's only roughly 1 in 100 cases.

- Your back could be a little sore for a day or two, but epidurals don't result in chronic back pain.

- After giving birth, you might have tingling or pins and needles down one leg. This happens in about one out of every 2000 cases. It may not be the epidural though, it's probably labor itself.

Spinal Block

A spinal block is a back injection that offers speedy anesthesia during surgery. It can also be used in conjunction with an epidural, to relieve labor pain quickly. You get a single injection of a numbing chemical that acts fast to help you feel comfortable. It's different from an epidural, in that it doesn't keep a plastic tube in place on your back so you can receive medication.

It's mostly used for C-sections, forceps deliveries, and all other surgical operations performed during pregnancy and childbirth. Believe it or not, it's the most popular option.

It takes about five minutes to carry out, and then another two to ten minutes for the anesthesia to start working. After the first minute, you'll feel warmth swiftly spread across your lower body and legs; it's comparable to stepping into a warm bath.

Following anesthesia, your and your baby's vital signs will be monitored.

Possible Reasons I Can't Have a Spinal

- Major blood coagulation abnormalities that make you bleed more than usual (including some anti-clotting medications).

- A back infection that affects the skin or tissue where a spinal would normally be placed.

- A severe sensitivity to the medicines used in spinal surgery (local anesthetics, opioids).

According to your doctor's assessment, the following conditions could make a spinal more difficult or dangerous but still feasible:

- Sepsis (Infection)

- Significant scoliosis or other modifications to the spine's form.

- A history of spinal surgery.

- Spina bifida

Side Effects and Risks

The likelihood of major issues for either mom or baby after receiving a spinal block is incredibly minimal. The key dangers and adverse effects of spinal blocks are listed here, and your anesthetist should go over them with you before inserting one.

The Epidural Information Card (2008), which you can find on the website of the Obstetric Anaesthetists' Association, served as the inspiration for the following list of spinal risks.

Risk/Side Effect	Chances
Accidental unconsciousness	1 in 100 000 women
Abscess	1 in 50 000 women
Haematoma	1 in 170 000 women
Meningitis	1 in 100 000 women
Nerve damage (numb patch on foot, or weak leg) lasting less than 6 months.	1 in 1000
Nerve damage (numb patch on foot, or weak leg) lasting over 6 months.	1 in 13 000

Paralysis or severe injury	1 in 250 000
Severe headache	1 in 500
Significant drop in bp	1 in 5
Spinal not working well enough for surgery	1 in 100

(Ridgeon, 2021)

Hydro—Water Birth

Water births take place in a warm water bath. Some women stay in the water during labor and then get out when it's time for delivery. Other women choose to deliver their babies in the water.

The theory is that after spending nine months in amniotic fluid, giving birth in a comparable environment is easier on the baby and less stressful for mom.

What Are the Risks?

- You or your child could contract an infection.

- It's possible for the umbilical cord to snap before your baby emerges from the water.

- The baby's temperature may be either too high or too low.

- Some water could go into your baby's lungs.

- Your baby might experience seizures or be unable to breathe.

What Precautions Can You Take?

If you're considering a water birth, find out early on in your pregnancy if the hospital offers the service. You also need to find out who's going to oversee your labor and delivery if they do. A midwife can help, but they will require medical support from a doctor.

If it's not offered at the hospital, you can either opt for a birthing center or your home.

Here are some things to look for:

- Your healthcare provider should be skilled and certified, so they're able to properly assist you with labor and delivery. But there should also always be a doctor present as a backup.

- The tub is clean and well-maintained.

- There are effective infection control procedures in place.

- While in the tub, you and your child are being appropriately monitored.

- There's an exit strategy in place to get you out of the tub as soon as your doctor, nurse, or midwife says so.

- The temperature of the water is always kept between 97 and 100 °F.

- You drink enough water throughout to avoid dehydration.

Are You a Good Candidate?

Don't attempt a water birth if:

- You have an infection.

- You have preeclampsia or diabetes.

- You're under 17 or over 35.

- You're pregnant with multiples.

- Your baby's breech.

- You're going into early labor.

- Your baby is large.

- There is severe meconium.

What Are the Costs?

It usually costs the same as a vaginal birth in a hospital, if it's covered by insurance. The tub may need to be rented, which might cost an additional $200 to $400.

Depending on your preferences, the cost of a tub or pool for a home birth might range from $65 to $500.

If a midwife or nurse-midwife comes to your home, they'll charge anywhere between $2,000 and $6,000. It's pretty much the same as a normal birth.

The midwife's fee may be covered by the facility if you give birth at a hospital or birthing center where they're employed. They charge anything between $3,000 and $4,000.

One major study conducted in 2020 found that women who completed a hypnobirthing program had significantly lower stress levels and pain ratings than those who did not. Also, there were reported benefits in terms of shorter labor, fewer interventions, and improved feelings of control over the birthing experience (University of Michigan, 2020).

Emotions in the Third Trimester

One thing that seems impossible during the third trimester, is getting a good night's sleep. Slumps in your mood may be caused by fatigue and sleep issues.

Anxieties about the impending birth, being a mother, or worrying about raising a human being can become very overwhelming.

On the positive side, nesting can be considered an emotional thing. When you suddenly feel the need to clean, arrange, and actually get ready for the baby, you are nesting. Not everybody experiences it, but for the moms who do, it can really feel like a positive experience.

At this stage in the pregnancy, we may start to interpret little things as big things, so it's important for us to know that not all pain is bad.

Braxton Hicks

Braxton hicks contractions are in all the movies. They're practice contractions that usually happen in the last few months of your pregnancy.

A Braxton hicks contraction might make your tummy feel hard. It will feel soft once again following the contraction.

Each contraction lasts between 30 and 60 seconds. They can occur throughout the day, but they might disappear when you workout and reappear when you relax.

Actual labor contractions are stronger and more frequent than Braxton Hicks. If you're a first-time mom, it might be challenging to distinguish between Braxton hicks and the real thing. Contact your midwife if you feel worried or anxious. Better safe than sorry.

What to Do if You Have Them

- Remain calm, do some breathing exercises, or go for a quick walk.

- A warm bath can ease some of the discomforts.

- Ask nicely for a shoulder or back rub from your partner.

- Stay hydrated and eat at regular intervals to maintain your energy levels.

Vaginal Bleeding in the Third Trimester

These are some potential reasons for vaginal bleeding in the second or third trimester:

- Uterine rupture: A rare but potentially fatal condition where the uterus ruptures along the scar from a previous C-section.

- Cervical issues: Like an infected or inflamed cervix or growths on the cervix

- Preterm labor: Light bleeding or spotting is common, as the fetal membranes can rupture (known as water breaking) before or during preterm labor.

- Placenta previa: The placenta typically develops at the top of the uterus during pregnancy. This is so that the cervix is unobstructed for delivery. Placenta previa occurs when the placenta is closer to the bottom of the uterus, partially or sometimes completely covering the cervix. In this position, the placenta often ruptures, leading to uncontrollable bleeding and the deprivation of essential nutrients and oxygen to the fetus.

- Placental abruption: This happens when the placenta detaches from the uterus before childbirth. It can result in serious bleeding and endanger both the mother and the unborn child's lives. There isn't medication or surgery to reconnect it, but prompt medical intervention may help raise the likelihood of a healthy birth after an abruption.

- Intrauterine fetal death: If the fetus remains in the body, the mother may have blood clots, infection, discomfort, fever, vomiting, diarrhea, and severe bleeding.

At the end of your pregnancy, you may notice light bleeding, usually mixed with mucus. It's normally pink in color, but it's called "bloody show." It's a sign that labor is starting.

Packing Your Bag for the Hospital

Once you've given birth, you'll be tired, disoriented, and hopefully on cloud nine. So your birthing partner or healthcare team should easily be able to find everything they need once the baby's born.

Being practical and having everything organized in different bags that you will bring in with you, is the best approach to preparing for a hospital stay:

A large bag (preferably a weekend bag)

A hospital bag for your baby

A separate bag for your birthing partner

To better keep track of the smaller items you've packed, you can use freezer bags or old shopping bags. Clear is better—this way you can label them.

We've got the bags down; let's get into their contents.

What to Pack

It's best to have your bag fully packed before you hit the 37-week mark. Pack the things you'll need later on in your stay first, so they're at the bottom of the bag. This will make finding everything so easy.

Main Bag

This will be your biggest bag; it should have space for 3 toiletry bags—your labor bag, post-birth bag, and baby's bag.

Checklist:

- Gadgets and chargers

- Breast pads and nipple cream

- Maternity pads

- Two light-weight dressing gowns (preferably dark in color)

- Two nightdresses (preferably with front button openings to facilitate skin-to-skin contact and breastfeeding)

- Three pairs of socks

- Five dark pairs of sweatpants (one will be in your post-birth bag)

- Three nursing bras

- A dark towel

- A change of clothes

Labor Bag

Put this bag at the very top of your main bag.

Checklist:

- A flannel

- A hand-fan

- Hair-ties

- A water bottle

- Massage oil

Post Birth Bag

This bag should include the things you'll need just after giving birth and for your first time in the bathroom post-birth.

Checklist:

- One pair of pants

- One nightdress

- Two maternity pads
- Flip flops (good for swollen feet)

Baby's Bag

Checklist:

- Ten nappies
- Four baby grows
- Four baby vests
- Five muslin cloths
- A blanket
- Two sets of hats and mitts
- Wet wipes
- Diaper cream

Birthing Partner's Bag

Checklist:

- Money
- A change of clothes
- Food and drinks
- Gadgets to pass the time (if need be)

- Power banks to charge their gadgets in case the hospital doesn't allow for them to use their power points.

After this month, things start to get a bit uncomfortable. Sometimes to the point where you start googling ways to induce labor. It might be too early for that, but it's never too early to start thinking about and weighing delivery options.

Your Baby's Development

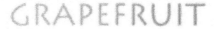

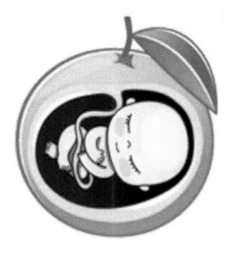

Congratulations on the beginning of the third trimester!

It may be a bit hard to celebrate, considering the back pain you might be experiencing. When your little one kicks at night, it probably keeps you awake, and if they don't kick during the day, you're probably not napping either.

Your child's head and your expanding uterus tend to rest on the sciatic nerve in the bottom part of your spine as baby prepares for delivery.

This may result in sciatica—a sharp, shooting pain, tingling, or numbness that begins in your buttocks and spreads down the back of your legs. The pain can at times be severe, only subsiding if the baby switches positions.

Your baby is measuring in at a whopping 15 inches long, and weighing in at 2.4 pounds. The same as a grapefruit. Your baby can now blink. That's just one of the many reflexes they've developed so far. Others include: hiccuping, sucking, coughing, and taking practice breaths.

Your baby has also started dreaming. When you move throughout the day, your baby becomes relaxed and falls asleep. Then, when it's your turn to sleep, baby is wide awake.

Chapter 8: Month Eight

Shower vs. Bath

A lot of women stick to showering once they find out they're pregnant because they're avoiding immersing themselves in tubs of hot water. But to a pregnant woman, a nice long bath probably sounds like a dream. It's so nice on the skin, and it can help alleviate some of those aches and pains.

It's perfectly safe to bathe, so long as you follow a few safety precautions.

As long as the water is warm, you're good to take a bath. Beyond that, what you have to think about is whether you're physically able to take that bath.

It can be challenging just getting into the tub, let alone reaching all the body parts that need washing and rinsing because of your expanding belly and declining energy. Keep in mind that you'll need to heave yourself out before you can towel off.

Hot Baths

As you near the end of your pregnancy, things start getting really uncomfortable, and you've probably said, "I want this baby out!" countless times

Naturally, you'll start to look up natural ways you can induce labor. One method that pops up quite a lot is taking a hot bath.

Unfortunately, hot baths are potentially dangerous to unborn babies, and there is no irrefutable proof to back up the theory that hot baths can jumpstart labor.

A baby may become distressed if the blood flow to their body is reduced. That can happen if the expectant mom sits in hot water. This is because the water can potentially raise your body temperature to over 101 °F. The temperature of the bath water should not exceed 98 °F. Also, sitting in the water for extended periods increases your risk of infection.

Speaking of infection…

Strep B

Group B strep is a common type of streptococcal bacteria found in the body—usually in the vagina or rectum. It's also referred to as GBS or strep B. Although carrying group B strep is mostly safe, it can occasionally infect a baby while you are in labor. The GBS infection can make your baby very ill, but with prompt treatment, most babies recover completely.

GBS causes sepsis, pneumonia, or meningitis. One in 14 newborns who recover from it will have a long-term disability of some kind. Tragically, 1 in 19 infants with an early-onset GBS infection passes away.

There are rare instances where it can affect the baby in utero. Those babies tend to fall ill within their first week of birth, and in other cases, it can take up to 3 months to manifest.

As GBS is not a sexually transmitted illness, the majority of carriers will not exhibit any symptoms.

During the third trimester of your pregnancy, you can request to undergo a group B strep screening test. Antibiotics can be prescribed to safeguard your baby if you have it during delivery.

At your doctor's appointment this month, you want to hear that the baby is finally head down. But there are actually an array of positions they could be in.

Presentation and Position of Baby for Delivery

Early on in your pregnancy, your baby moves around freely in the womb because there's an abundance of space. However, as they grow, they have less wiggle room.

What Is Fetal Position?

Fetal positioning refers to how your unborn child, or fetus, is laid out in the womb, whether that means on its back, with its head down, or any other way. The *fetal position* refers to the traditional curled-up baby position.

With the head down, a curved spine, and the arms and legs drawn close to the body, it resembles the shape of a C. Your baby will stretch, kick, and move around from time to time, but this is usually the position they'll choose to stay in most of the time.

It's the most comfortable position for your baby in the womb and for a while after birth. It actually helps your baby get into the optimum position for birth and reduces the possibility of difficulties.

Types of Fetal Positioning for Birth

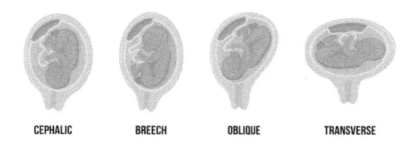

CEPHALIC   BREECH   OBLIQUE   TRANSVERSE

Most babies can position themselves head down by 36 weeks for an easy exit. Others decide they're completely at ease and have no intention of leaving.

Breech position

Just 3 to 4% of babies born at full term choose to remain in the breech position, head up and bottom down. There are different types, and they all raise the possibility that you might need a C-section (*Movement and Positions during Labour*, n.d.)

- **Complete breech**: Baby's knees are bent, and their feet are close to their bottom, which is near the birth canal.

- **Footling breech**: Baby has one or both legs near or in the birth canal.

- **Frank breech**: Baby is shaped like a V, with its feet close to its head, legs up, and bottom near the birth canal.

Oblique position

Oblique means your baby is sitting diagonally or is slanted across the womb. It's quite uncommon, but not impossible.

Because the head isn't properly aligned with the birth canal, there is a higher risk of umbilical cord compression during delivery. If the umbilical cord enters the birth canal first, pressure from the head may compress the cord, impeding blood flow and creating a crisis.

If medical personnel can't turn your baby into a head-down position, you might need to have a C-section.

Occiput Anterior

This is the ideal fetal position for delivery. Baby is feet up, head down, facing your back, with their back resting against your tummy. The back of their head is close to your pubic bone, and they can exit the birth canal with ease.

It's also called the "vertex position" or "cephalic position."

There's really no *easy* way to give birth, but this position makes it easier for your baby to descend and for you to deliver. Your baby has the best chance of passing through the birth canal this way.

Occiput Posterior

This position is almost identical to the OA, with the exception that the baby is now facing your belly rather than your back. Other names for it are the back-to-back and sunny-side-up positions.

Your baby can't tuck their chin down to easily pass through the birth canal in this position. Labor could take longer if your baby is unable to turn over. A C-section might be recommended by your doctor for safety.

Transverse Position

When a baby is transverse, they're in the fetal position while resting sideways across the womb. In this position, you never know whether their back, shoulders, hands, or feet could be closest to the birth canal.

The most dangerous thing about this position is that the placenta could be damaged during delivery or when trying to turn the baby over. Your doctor will make the call on whether a C-section is the most prudent course of action.

Cesarean Section

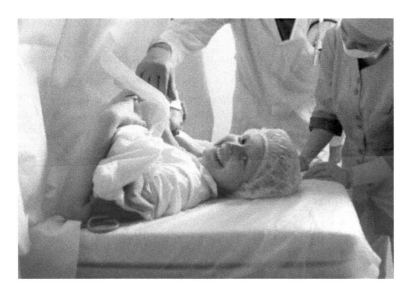

A cesarean section is a surgical operation that's employed to deliver a baby when a vaginal delivery can't be performed safely. It's usually done in an emergency, but it can also be an elective surgery that's scheduled ahead of time. It has a somewhat longer recovery time and a higher risk than a vaginal delivery.

Reasons to Have One

- Breech presentation

- **Cephalopelvic disproportion (CPD)**: Your baby's head or body is too large to fit through your pelvis, or your pelvis is too small to birth an average-sized baby.

- Expecting multiples

- **Health issues**: Labor can exacerbate health issues like cardiovascular disease. If you have a venereal disease like herpes, vaginal birth is not an option.

- **Obstruction**: You might need a C-section if you have a large uterine fibroid, a pelvic fracture, or if you're expecting a child with any congenital abnormalities.

- Placenta previa

- Previous C-section

- Transverse lie

What Are the Risks?

- Fetal injury

- Problems with general anesthesia

- Abnormalities of future placentas

- A weakened uterine wall

- Damage to the bladder or bowel

- Embolism

- Hemorrhage

- Infection

Recovery

You'll start to feel the pain from the incisions when the anesthetic wears off. It creeps up on you at first and then becomes a bit more pronounced, but it's nothing painkillers can't fix. Also, it might be difficult to take deep breaths, and you may feel gassy. For the first few days after surgery, make sure you have assistance getting out of bed from an adult. C-section moms usually stay in the hospital for up to three days after giving birth.

It can take anywhere from four to six weeks to fully recover. Medical professionals advise abstaining from stairs, lifting, and strenuous activity, for several weeks. So that you can relax and heal nicely, ask your friends, family, or partner to help with errands. This includes driving.

For those six weeks, you can anticipate cramps, bleeding, and some discomfort near the incision. For pain, over-the-counter painkillers like acetaminophen or ibuprofen can help. For at least six weeks—or until your doctor gives the all-clear—avoid engaging in any sexual activity.

As your uterine lining sheds following the procedure, you will have vaginal discharge—called "lochia." It starts out crimson and progressively turns yellow. If you encounter severe bleeding or a bad odor coming from your discharge, make sure to contact your healthcare professional right away. Use sanitary pads rather than tampons until all of your bleeding has stopped.

Vaginal Birth After Delivery

A lot of women who've had C-sections think about the possibility of vaginal delivery in their subsequent pregnancies. The odds of having a vaginal birth after a cesarean (VBAC) are higher if you meet the following requirements:

- Your first C-section was not an emergency one.

- You're not carrying multiples.

- Your pelvis is not too narrow to support a baby of typical size.

- Your doctor made a small transverse incision.

Is It Safe?

When you've had surgery on your uterus, it leaves a scar. Doctors fear that the strain of labor can cause that scar to rupture.

But after years of research, it was found that 60% to 80% of women who had cesarean births also had healthy vaginal births in their subsequent pregnancies. The National Institute of Child Health and Human Development released figures that lend credence to the safety of VBAC. They found that 75% of VBAC attempts are successful. (*Vaginal Birth after Cesarean (VBAC): Facts, Safety & Risks*, 2021)

Am I at Risk of a Uterine Rupture?

The probability of a ruptured uterus after a previous C-section with a horizontal (transverse) cut is around 0.9%, or little less than 1 in 100, according to the American College of Obstetricians and Gynecologists (2021).

Risks associated with a ruptured uterus include:

- Damage to the bladder

- Infection

- Blood clots

- Blood loss

- Hysterectomy

Natural vs. C-Section

Natural Pros

- Vaginal births often need shorter recuperation and hospital stays.

- The dangers of major surgery, like hemorrhaging, scarring, infections, reactions to anesthesia, and intense pain, are often avoided with vaginal births. Also, moms are able to start breastfeeding earlier because they've avoided surgery.

- A baby who is born vaginally will be able to interact with their mother more quickly since she can start breastfeeding right away.

- The muscles used in a vaginal delivery are more likely to press out the fluid in a newborn's lungs, which is good since it reduces the likelihood of breathing difficulties at birth.

Natural Cons

- A vaginal delivery is a long, physically taxing process. First-time mothers often have active labor for four to eight hours on average.

- The skin and surrounding tissues of the vagina are in danger of stretching and rupturing once the fetus passes through the birth canal. Stitches may be needed for severe tears and stretching. The pelvic muscles that regulate bowel and urinary movements may become weak or suffer an injury as a result of the stretching and tearing.

- Studies found that women who gave birth vaginally were more likely to develop pelvic organ prolapse, which is when one or more organs drop into the pelvis. They were also at risk of developing urinary incontinence, which causes urine to leak when a person laughs, sneezes, or coughs.

- Moreover, the perineum, which is located between the vagina and the anus, may continue to hurt indefinitely after a vaginal delivery.

- Newborns can sustain injuries during the birth process itself, resulting in a bruised scalp or a fractured collarbone. It mostly happens if a woman has had a long labor or if the baby is large.

Cesarean Pros

- If a woman has extreme anxiety around giving birth vaginally, she may decide to have a C-section and save herself from a negative experience.

- Women who undergo C-sections are less likely to get pelvic organ prolapse and suffer incontinence.

- Compared to natural labor, a surgical birth can be planned in advance, making it convenient and predictable.

- A C-section can save both mom and baby's lives in emergency situations.

Cesarean Cons

- The average hospital stay following a C-section is two to four days. Moreover, there may be increased abdominal pain and discomfort during the healing time.

- Due to the various potential complications, women are three times more likely to die with a cesarean delivery than with a natural birth.

- A woman is more likely to get a C-section in the future if she has already had one.

- Infants delivered through C-section may be more susceptible to respiratory issues both at birth and later in life.

- There is a slight possibility that a baby could be cut by the scalpel during a surgery and get hurt.

EGGPLANT

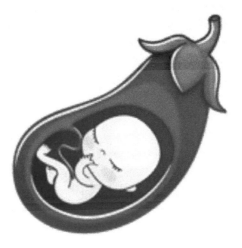

This month, your uterus is just inches above your belly button, so some of your organs up THERE are really feeling it. It's crowded up there. This means you'll experience some shortness of breath as your lungs and diaphragm are a bit squished.

Something to look out for is Braxton hicks. Chances are, you're starting to experience them now.

Baby is weighing in at 3.5–4 pounds and measuring in at 16–17 inches. They're about as big as an eggplant. Baby is quickly running out of legroom and is now in the fetal position. There's fat accumulation under baby's skin now so they're no longer translucent. Baby is hard at work and continue to hone their skills in breathing and sucking.

Chapter 9: Month Nine

Finally! Baby could come any day now. You're probably hoping it's sooner rather than later. By now, you've probably got a birth plan in place, but it's time to start considering what could happen if you can't wait for nature to take its course.

It's also a good time to give more thought to how you'd like to look after your baby once they're here.

Planned Induction

It's always best to let nature take its course, but there are instances where nature could use a push. If healthcare providers are under the impression that delivering sooner is the best course of action, they'll suggest an induction.

Possible Reasons for Induction

- When the due date has come and gone and there are no signs of labor (post-term pregnancy).

- When your water breaks and labor doesn't start (premature rupture of membranes).

- Getting a uterine infection.

- Fetal growth restriction.

- When there is insufficient amniotic fluid surrounding the baby (oligohydramnios).

- Having diabetes, type 2 or gestational.

- Elevated blood pressure.

- Placental abruption.

- Medical conditions like obesity or kidney disease.

Elective Labor Induction

Elective labor induction is usually for convenience—there's no medical emergency attached to it.

To lower the baby's risk of health issues, a medical professional will verify that the gestational age of the baby is at least 39 weeks or older before inducing labor.

Recent studies have led to the provision of labor induction for women with low-risk pregnancies at 39 to 40 weeks. Starting labor early minimizes a number of risks, including those related to stillbirth, macrosomia (refers to growth beyond 8 pounds 13 ounces, regardless of gestational age), and the development of high blood pressure if the pregnancy progresses. The decision to induce labor should be a joint one between the expectant mother and her healthcare practitioners.

Risks

There are instances in which a woman shouldn't undergo labor induction. If you've had a C-section, or significant uterine surgery, placenta previa, or if your baby is breech or transverse, it might not be an option for you.

Other dangers associated with inducing labor include:

- **Bleeding after delivery**: The likelihood that the uterine muscles won't adequately contract after giving birth (uterine atony) increases when labor is induced. This can cause substantial bleeding after birth.

- **Failed induction**: If the proper induction techniques don't result in a vaginal delivery after 24 or more hours, the induction is deemed unsuccessful and might result in a C-section.

- **Infection**: Certain labor induction techniques, like rupturing the membranes may raise the danger of infection for both mom and baby.

- **Low fetal heart rate**: Oxytocin and prostaglandin (the medications used to induce labor) cause irregular or excessive contractions, which might reduce the baby's oxygen supply and drop its heart rate.

- **Uterine rupture**: These occur when the uterus tears along the scar line from a prior significant uterine surgery. The complications can be life-threatening, so in order to avoid that, an emergency C-section will be performed and the uterus removed if necessary.

What to Expect

Induction involves a number of steps, but depending on how you respond to each one, your doctor may not have to follow through with the next ones.

Cervical Ripening

Your doctor will need to start the ripening process if your cervix doesn't show any signs of softening, opening, or thinning to allow your baby to exit the uterus and enter the birth canal. The doctor will usually do this by applying topical prostaglandin to your cervix. It can come in the form of a gel or a vaginal suppository. A few hours after that, your cervix will be checked. Ripening is usually enough to initiate labor and contractions.

Sometimes the prostaglandin does ripen the cervix, but contractions still don't start. In that case, your doctor will move on to the subsequent steps.

If you've had any previous uterine surgery, you won't be given prostaglandin in an attempt to avoid uterine rupture. Your doctor might opt for a graduated dilator or catheter with an inflating balloon.

Membrane Stripping

Your doctor may be able to get labor started by swiping their finger across the delicate membranes connecting the amniotic sac if it's still intact. This is supposed to encourage the uterus to release prostaglandin, which should soften the cervix and allow contractions to start.

Although it isn't intended to break your water, it can happen, and it does tend to be painful.

Membrane Rupturing

Your doctor may artificially rupture the membranes to kick-start your contractions if your cervix has already started to dilate and efface but your water hasn't broken.

This involves manually bursting the amniotic sac with a device that resembles a long, sharp crochet hook. It can be uncomfortable, but it shouldn't hurt.

Pitocin

If none of the previous steps took effect and labor hasn't started, your doctor will progressively administer the drug Pitocin via an IV to trigger or intensify contractions. Pitocin is a synthetic version of the hormone oxytocin. Although you won't have anything to compare it to if this is your first child, Pitocin-induced contractions are stronger, more regular, and more frequent than natural ones. They start as quickly as 30 minutes after the Pitocin is administered. If you know you'd like an epidural, talk to your doctor about starting it while you receive Pitocin so that it will be ready when labor actually begins.

Breast vs. Bottle

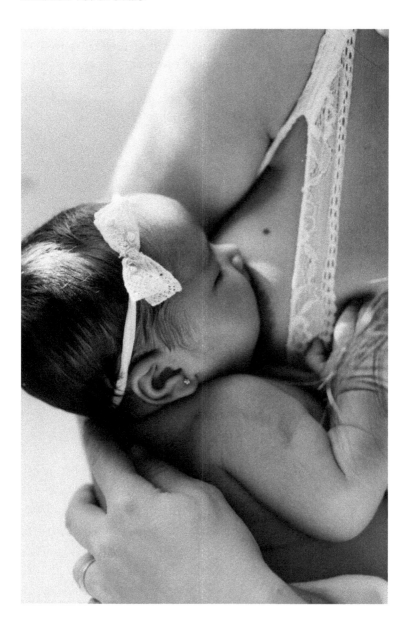

The feeding method that has the most benefits for both mother and child is breastfeeding. Health experts advise that babies should consume only breast milk for the first four to six months of their lives and then stick with it as a major source of nutrition until they are at least one to two years old.

Baby formula is designed to provide newborns with a nutritious supply of sustenance. There are several different formulas available for infants from the day they're born. The nutrients, calories, taste, digestibility, and price of infant formulas vary. There are options for almost every situation. Whether your baby is lactose intolerant, has a milk protein allergy, or has a metabolic condition, you will be able to find a formula for them.

At the end of the day, how and what you choose to feed your baby is your decision. All babies need to be fed.

Here are some of the benefits and drawbacks of both breastfeeding and formula feeding.

Breastfeeding vs. Formula Feeding Pros and Cons

Breastfeeding Pros

- All the nutrients that newborns need to grow and develop are in breast milk.

- The antibodies in breast milk help keep your baby healthy.

- Babies who are breastfed have a lower risk of developing respiratory illnesses.

- Breastfeeding can help your infant avoid health issues like allergies, eczema, ear infections, and gastrointestinal issues.

- It's easier for breastfeeding mothers to shed weight after giving birth.

- Breastfeeding possibly lowers the risk of diabetes and various cancers.

Breastfeeding Cons

- Discomfort in the nipples and breasts. Very common in the first week. Also, learning how to nurse can take a couple of weeks.

- Breast heaviness or engorgement.

- Obstructed milk ducts

- Insufficient milk to meet the baby's needs.

Formula Pros

- There's more freedom of movement because anyone can feed your baby.

- You can get away with longer intervals between feeds, because babies take longer to digest formula.

- You can actually measure and be sure of how much your baby consumes.

- Your baby will be able to bond with more family members during feeds.

Formula Cons

- Babies are not as well protected against Infections, illnesses, and disorders on formula.

- You have to properly mix and prepare the formula, while ensuring the temperature is right.

- All the accessories that come with bottle-feeding can be pricey.

- Babies may experience constipation and gas as a result of the formula.

Breastfeeding Myths

Baby won't consume enough milk

Virtually all women can produce adequate milk for their babies, regardless of breast or nipple size or shape.

The best way to keep your supply going is through early and frequent feedings and ongoing skin-to-skin contact.

When you've got a good supply going, the amount of breast milk you produce will precisely correspond with your baby's needs. Your body generates more milk as you breastfeed.

Your partner may feel left out

There are so many ways for partners to get close to the baby, and many ways for them to support you too, for instance:

- They can bring you water or snacks while you're feeding.

- Have skin-to-skin contact with the baby.

- Cuddling the baby.

- Changing diapers.

- Burping.

- Bathing the baby.

It makes your breasts sag

Your breasts won't sag because of breastfeeding. The ligaments supporting your breasts can swell because of pregnancy hormones. They also just may appear to sag as you age.

You can prevent it by wearing bras that fit properly.

You have to stop at 6 months

There is no stipulation on when you should stop breastfeeding.

The World Health Organization suggests that you (*Breastfeeding - Common Myths*, 2022):

- Breastfeed exclusively for the first six months.

- Continue breastfeeding while feeding supplemental foods, until two years and even beyond.

Your Baby's Development

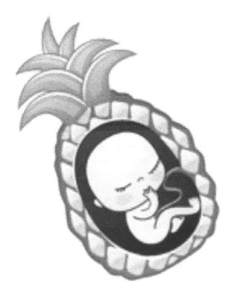

PINEAPPLE

As hormones that loosen and soften joints begin to take effect before labor, this last month may bring more joint flexibility and pelvic pain. You'll also just be experiencing more and more of the same discomfort you've had for the past couple of months.

Baby is measuring in at 18–19 inches, and weighs in at roughly 6 pounds. They're about the size of a pineapple. They won't grow much more now; otherwise, you'd burst. Baby is pretty much fully developed and ready to go. They just need a couple more weeks inside so their digestive system can catch up with the rest of them.

Baby is probably eavesdropping on you because of their sharpened sense of hearing. They're also moving lower into your pelvis... Fun...

Trimester 4:

The Stork Has Arrived

Chapter 10: Labor

Signs You're Going Into Labor Soon

Your back hurts

Most pregnant women experience back pain the entire time. But, if the pain intensifies or is central to your lower back, it may indicate that you are going through *back labor*, which happens when the baby is head down and facing forward. According to the Cleveland Clinic (n.d.), up to 32% of newborns are in this position in the beginning stages of labor.

Your baby's face is usually pressed against your spine as they go down into the birth canal, but when a baby's skull is on your spine, it can hurt. You'll feel the pain in your abdomen, but it'll mostly be localized in your back.

Some pregnant women may also have back pain-like contractions or back pain that radiates to or from their back. This may not be back labor, but any severe back pain may be an indication that labor is about to start.

You see a bloody show

For the entirety of your pregnancy, your cervix stays closed. It's clogged up with mucus that works to protect your baby from infection,

Once you go into labor, it's not needed anymore, so as labor progresses, the cervix starts to soften, dilate, and efface in anticipation of delivery, which causes the plug to make its way out. The mucus is expelled as a blob or like discharge, and it can weigh up to 1–2 tablespoons and measure as much as 2 inches.

As your cervix continues to dilate and efface, microscopic blood vessels rupture along its surface, tainting the mucus and giving it a brown (from old blood) or pink hue. Labor could start hours, days, or even weeks after you see it.

Losing your mucus plug is usually a sign that labor is starting, but keep in mind that it can be displaced gradually over time, so you won't always notice it. If you've still got it, or even trace amounts of it, it can indicate that delivery could happen soon.

Your water breaks

The amniotic sac doesn't always rupture prior to the onset of contractions. In reality, many women start their labor well before their water breaks. Also, the experience looks and feels different for everyone. For some, it's more of a little leak than a large gush.

But, if your sac does rupture on its own, it usually indicates that labor is about to start, if it hasn't already. About 90% of full-term pregnancies, 37 weeks or more along, experience spontaneous labor within 24 hours of the water breaking. Those that don't are likely to undergo an induction because after the amniotic sac has ruptured, the risk of infection increases (*Water Breaking: Understand This Sign of Labor*, 2019).

Timing Contractions

What Do They Feel Like?

Your womb thickens during a contraction before relaxing. A lot of women describe them as a feeling like severe period pains.

They will likely get longer, intensify, and become more frequent as labor progresses. Muscles constrict, and discomfort rises with a contraction; your belly actually becomes harder while it's happening. The hardness will subside as the muscles relax and the pain eases.

The contractions are lowering your baby and widening your cervix so they can go through the birth canal.

When to Start Timing

You can determine whether you are in actual labor by timing your contractions.

When your contractions start to happen closer together, and get stronger, start timing them. The best way to get an indication of their frequency is to start by timing three in a row. You can use your phone or a stopwatch.

Once they're happening at least every five minutes, and lasting a minute at a time, you should start making your way to where you're going to deliver.

What if I Don't Make It Out of the House in Time?

In the unlikely event that you are unable to reach the hospital in time, commit this piece of advice to memory so that you are ready.

If you're genetically predisposed to giving birth faster and you're aware of it, time your contractions from the beginning and go to the hospital just in case. If you spontaneously feel the urge to push after a short labor period, and you aren't at home, don't panic. Many babies have been born in moving vehicles. Even though it's unlikely, being ready for an emergency delivery at home could curb your worry and make you feel comfortable knowing that you can manage the situation.

A few years ago, the American College of Nurse-Midwives (ACNM) started a program called "Giving Birth in Place" to inform individuals on how to prepare for emergency deliveries at home.

They say it's best to stay where you are if you've got a strong feeling you won't make it to the hospital. It's recommended that you assemble a delivery-ready supply kit for emergency situations. The items should be stored out of reach of kids and animals in a waterproof bag. The following should be packed in:

- A bag of extra-large underpads with a plastic back to shield sheets from bodily fluids.

- Bulb syringe in a baby-safe size. It must be made of soft plastic, and be an ear syringe so it can fit in baby's nose.

- A chemical cold pack.

- A small isopropyl alcohol bottle.

- 12 maternity pads.

- One pack of large cotton balls.

- Sharp, clean scissors (to cut the cord).

- A box of single-use latex or plastic gloves.

- White shoelaces (to tie the cord).

- A hot water bottle (for the baby).

- Ibuprofen or acetaminophen.

- An antibacterial liquid hand sanitizer or a little bar of soap

- Six diapers.

Stages of Labor

Stage one

Your contractions intensify, and your cervix dilates to a diameter of 10 cm.

Stage two

You'll experience painful contractions, and eventually, the need to push. You'll receive instructions from your midwife on how to control your breathing during contractions. It is at this point that your baby will be delivered.

Stage three

After giving birth to your child, you push the placenta out. Stage three is also called "the afterbirth." Your midwife or doctor may offer you a shot to help you along.

Should I Shave?

The times have definitely changed. People are less worried about the little things. So a bit of hair down there isn't going to shock or worry your doctor.

The medical staff's role is to ensure that both you and the baby have a safe birth. They have no concerns or worries regarding the appearance of your perineum.

Hospitals used to shave women in preparation for delivery, but that's changed, and it's now recommended that you don't shave at all. At least not past 36 weeks gestation.

The belief was that shaving would prevent infection, but as time goes on and medicine advances, there's been evidence of a slight increase in infection after shaving.

Try not to worry about judgment; the chances of you facing any are slim to none. If you really must groom, opt for a wax or any other method that doesn't involve a razor.

Breath Techniques

Learn and practice regulated breathing techniques for labor pain management before you go into labor. By focusing on your breathing, you can keep your oxygen levels high, relax your muscles and mind, and get some relief from the discomfort.

Before giving birth, practice the breathing exercises below if you haven't already studied specialized breathing methods at a birthing class:

- **Belly breathing**

Try belly breathing when labor is still early. When you breathe in, let your belly expand outward; when you exhale, let your belly relax downward.

Place one hand right below your ribs on your abdomen, and the other on your chest.

Inhale deeply through your nose, allowing your abdomen to push your hand away. Your chest should remain still.

Put your lips together and exhale like you're whistling. Use the hand that is placed on your tummy to force all the air out.

During or in between contractions, do this exercise. Breathe slowly each time.

- **Pant-pant-blow breathing**

Belly breathing will be harder as labor progresses, so exhale six times per minute in a "pant-pant-blow" sequence as your contractions get stronger.

At the beginning of your contraction, inhale deeply through your nose.

Exhale by doing two brief blows followed by one longer blow. It sounds like "hee-hee-hooooo." You see it in movies.

It should take about 10 seconds to breathe in and out like this.

Keep breathing like this until the contraction stops.

Fetal and Internal Monitoring

Your doctor will want to examine your baby's health both during pregnancy and labor. They monitor baby by checking the heart rate and other vital signs.

There are two ways doctors monitor babies. On the outside of your tummy (external monitoring) and on the inside (internal monitoring):

- **External monitoring**: A fetoscope is a specialized instrument used to monitor the baby's heartbeat. It's a stethoscope with a distinct shape. The baby can also be monitored using a doppler.

- **Internal monitoring**: The medical staff attach an electrode onto the baby's head while in utero.

Your midwife keeps an eye on your baby's heartbeat during labor so they can identify any indication of trouble as soon as possible. The range of a healthy heart rate is 110 to 160 beats per minute.

The healthcare team might also make use of:

Intermittent Monitoring

Being monitored at regular intervals throughout labor.

The midwife may use a fetoscope or a doppler. She'll place one of the instruments on your belly to hear baby's heartbeat. She'll do so every 15 minutes in the first stage of labor and every five minutes in the second.

Should there be any concerns about you or your baby, they will start electronic monitoring.

Electronic Fetal Monitoring (EFM)

Continuously keep an eye on the two of you...

Medical staff will put electrodes on your belly. The electrodes are attached to a large machine that continually prints waves that signify your contractions and the baby's heartbeat. Instead of paper, some machines display everything on a screen.

Or, with your permission, they might place the electrodes directly on to baby's head so they can monitor the heartbeat.

EFM is usually used when you're past 42 weeks gestation, or when you ask for an epidural. It also gets recommended if:

- Your temperature or blood pressure are high.

- There are concerns about your baby's growth or heartbeat.

- Your waters are sparse, your waters break more than 24 hours before labor, or they are stained with meconium or blood.

- You're being induced, you're on oxytocin, or your labor's lasting longer than 8 hours.

Fetal Blood Sampling

A small blood sample is taken by an obstetrician to determine baby's heart rate.

If they're worried about your baby's heartbeat, your healthcare team will ask an obstetrician to check, and the doctor might advise you to get a blood sample. They will need your permission before they can do anything.

You tilt or sleep on your left side with your right leg lifted, and then your doctor will put a speculum in your vagina, make a little cut on your infant's scalp, and then get a drop or two of blood.

They're looking at the acid and oxygen levels in the blood sample. These results can indicate how well your baby is responding to labor.

If it's normal, you get to stay in labor. If it's not and your baby's in distress, your obstetrician could advise that they deliver your child right away.

What Positions Are Best for Labor?

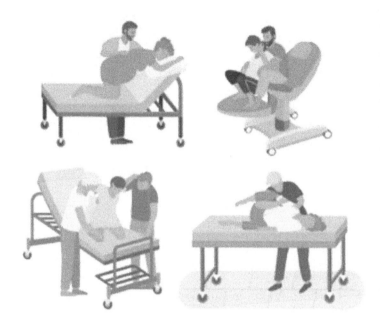

The immediate picture you have in your mind of a woman giving birth is her reclining in a hospital bed. In reality, women move about a lot during labor and change positions as their labor develops and the baby shifts positions.

Moving, maintaining balance, and shifting positions can:

- Help you determine your ideal birthing position.

- Help the baby move down.

- Shorten labor time

- Reduce discomfort.

- Help you to cope.

- Give you a sense of control over your labor.

Good Positions to Try

- Straddling a chair.

- Standing and leaning against something.

- Seated and leaning against a table.

- Standing and leaning on a birth ball that is perched on a bed.

- Hugging a birth ball while in a squatting position.

- Getting on all fours and kneeling.

- Sitting and bouncing softly on a birth ball.

- Kneeling over the back of your bed, or kneeling and leaning against your birth partner for support.

If you can, try to walk around as much as you can. You can try to maintain motion by shifting your weight from one foot to the other or by rolling your pelvis if you start to feel fatigued or your contractions become more intense.

Your birth partner will be able to give you massages or stroke your back in some of the positions listed above. It will help you release some endorphins, which might help a little with the pain.

Don't forget to take breaks when necessary, and don't give a second thought to how you look or sound during any of this. Medical staff have seen it all before and then some.

What Can Your Birthing Partner Do?

Birth partners can enhance the experience and make a woman feel supported while in labor. Here are some pointers on how to be a fantastic one:

- **Be prepared and ready**

    Birth partners need to be fully prepared and on standby.

    If a birth plan is in place, it should be discussed at length and in advance with the mom-to-be. A partner can learn about what to anticipate by taking birth classes together with the mom.

    Ask mom if there's anything in particular that can be done to help her during labor and delivery. Ask about the things you shouldn't involve yourself with, as well. Know your boundaries; if there are aspects of the delivery you would prefer not to participate in directly, let it be known in advance.

    If there's anything you're not confident with yet, make sure you learn and practice it in time for the birth.

- **Provide good company**

During the early stages of labor, especially, keep mom company, ensure she's happy, and try to pass the time together.

You might be able to spend time together walking, watching TV, listening to music, or reading. Literally, anything to get her mind off the discomfort.

Do anything and everything you can to help her feel more at ease. She might want help taking a bath or shower. You can get her things to help soothe her, or help her maneuver that.

Look after yourself too, and take breaks when you need to. Choose comfortable clothes and pack snacks for yourself so you can stay in peak shape.

- **Provide practical support**

You can help in so many little ways. Driving mom to the hospital, carrying the bags, and getting her checked into the birthing suite or hospital.

Once you're in the labor and delivery ward you can help her get comfortable in the bed, help her turn around if need be. A refreshment and a back rub would also go down really nicely.

If you've opted for a home birth, you can help set everything up. Then on the day, you can offer refreshments and keep the family updated with how things are going.

This step hinges on you, knowing well in advance how everything needs to happen.

- **Advocate for her**

  You might need to let the midwife or doctor know what mom needs because you know her best. Help her communicate her wishes to them. Also, you might need to keep her updated on all new information that comes from the medical staff.

  Even if she chooses something completely off from her birth plan, you should still support her choices.

- **Be flexible**

  You can do all the preparation in the world, but you'll need to adapt to whatever's working or not working throughout labor because no two labors are the same. It's possible that everything can go as planned, but it's also possible that an urgent medical issue could occur and change how the labor progresses.

  Whatever happens, try to let mom know and keep encouraging and reassuring her. She will feel less powerless and a bit more in control of the situation.

  You might have to make very important decisions at the drop of a hat, or you might have to wait really long for her labor to progress. Be ready to be flexible and ride the wave of the day.

Chapter 11: Delivery

The hope for all deliveries is that they're straightforward. In the event that things don't go exactly according to plan, you should have some knowledge of the types of interventions that are used and how they affect you. That way you'll always be making informed decisions.

What's an Episiotomy?

Your vagina and perineum are incredibly elastic; they're able to expand to accommodate the birth of your child.

On occasion, a member of your healthcare team may need to make a cut in your perineum to widen the opening at your vagina. This is an episiotomy. It gets sewn up once the baby is born.

Episiotomies are only performed when necessary, so they don't happen for every labor.

They're done mostly to stop tearing or in situations where moms just need a bit of help. They're most likely in vaginal births.

Other Reasons for Episiotomies

- Baby's in distress. Their heart rate is either too fast or too slow; this could mean that they aren't getting enough oxygen.

- Your baby's breech.

- Your baby's bigger than average.

- Your doctor plans on using forceps or a ventouse.

- Your doctor advises that you have a quick labor because you have medical issues, like a heart condition.

- You've been exerting yourself for a while and are worn out.

- It's required to stop a third-degree tear from happening (a third-degree tear is a perineum muscular tear that also impacts the anus muscles).

Recovery

Keeping It Clean

To clean your perineum, use only warm water. Avoid rubbing it when cleaning. Witch hazel and salt are assumed to support the acceleration of wound healing, but there isn't any scientific proof of this. However, if you want to use them, there's no harm in doing so.

Wear underwear that's made of breathable materials, like cotton. Put on comfy, loose clothing while you're healing, because tight clothing may hurt you.

Clean your hands
- both before and after using the restroom.

- before and after cleaning your wound.

- when swapping out your pad.

If you live with young children, washing up and being clean are extremely important because they could be carrying an illness like Group A strep that could spread to your wound. Once it enters the bloodstream, things can become quite serious.

Going to the Loo

Wash your perineum each and every time you're done in the restroom. Put warm water around your vaginal area as well. Pouring warm water on your outer vagina while you urinate might also lessen the stinging sensation from the urine.

Lean forward toward your knees while urinating. This will assist in diverting urine away from the wound.

Your First Bowel Movement

After giving birth, your back passage and bottom may feel a little sore.

When you're ready to poop, your first instinct might be to worry about your stitches. You don't have to; pooping won't make you lose your stitches or open your incision. You can take steps to make pooping more bearable.

As you poop, place a clean pad at the side of your incision and gently push. This may relieve some of the pressure you'll feel on the wound.

Wipe gently from front to back. This lessens the chance of bacteria infecting the wound.

Do your best to avoid constipation. Drink plenty of water and consume foods high in fiber.

Pain Management

Paracetamol is safe to take, and it works well in relieving pain. If you're breastfeeding, you can take two 500-milligram pills every six hours.

Diclofenac pills or suppositories are also really good. Suppositories offer pain relief for a longer time and can be inserted once every 18 hours. If you're unsure about how to put them in, you can ask your midwife.

Aspirin can't be taken if you're breastfeeding.

If paracetamol and diclofenac don't work, call your doctor so they can check and see if it's infected.

Infection indicators:

- redness

- a yellow or green discharge

- extreme pain

Let the medical team know if you're breastfeeding so they can prescribe pain medication that's not harmful to your breastfed baby.

Forceps and Vacuum Births

Forceps and vacuum births are also called "assisted births." Your healthcare team only makes use of them when labor has stalled, or when delivery is about to end but is not progressing, and the health of you or your baby is at risk from an extended labor.

Forceps look like metal salad utensils that the doctor can use to guide your baby out of the birth canal by grasping them while they're still inside. A ventouse is a suction cup used to get your baby out of the birth canal. They don't happen too often, but they can be a helpful alternative to a cesarean.

What Happens?

Before anything happens, your healthcare team will need your permission.

If you haven't already had an epidural, you'll get a local anesthetic to numb your vagina and perineum. If your doctor has concerns, you might be taken to an operating room so that, if necessary, you can get a C-section.

To widen the vaginal orifice, your doctor might do an episiotomy. Your birth partner might still be able to cut the cord if they want to, because once your baby's out, they are placed on your tummy.

Forceps

Forceps are curved so they can fit around a baby's head. Doctors gently wrap the baby's head in the forceps, which are joined together at the handle. The doctor then carefully pulls while you push during a contraction.

There are lots of different types. Some are made specifically to turn the baby into the proper position for birth. For example, if the baby's lying to one side (occipito-lateral position) or facing up (occipito-posterior position).

Ventouse

The suction cup is attached to a tube that connects to a suction device. The baby's head is firmly supported by the cup, and then the doctor gently pulls the baby while you push during a contraction.

Forceps are usually suggested over a suction cup, especially if you're giving birth before 36 weeks. It's because forceps are less likely to harm the baby's head while it's still soft.

Why Would I Need One?

- You've got an underlying health condition like hypertension, so you're advised not to push.

- Your baby's heart rate is worrying.

- Your baby's in an awkward position.

- Your baby's energy is dwindling, and might be in distress.

- When you deliver a premature baby vaginally, forceps can assist in shielding your baby's head from your perineum.

Potential Risks

For you:

- **Anal incontinence**: After delivery, anal incontinence can occur, especially if there is a third- or fourth-degree tear. These tears are very common with assisted deliveries.

- **Urinary incontinence**: Urinary incontinence after delivery is quite common. It happens a lot after a forceps or ventouse delivery. You can prevent it with physiotherapy and pelvic floor exercises.

- **Higher risk of blood clots**: Blood clots in the pelvic or leg veins are more likely to occur after an assisted birth. You can avoid them by being physically active after birth. You can also wear anti-clot stockings, or your doctor might give you heparin injections.

- **Third and fourth-degree tears**: These kinds of tears affect:

  - 3 out of every 100 women giving birth naturally

- 4 out of every 100 women in a ventouse delivery

- 8–12 out of every 100 women in forceps delivery

For baby:

- A ventouse cup mark is left on a baby's head. It's called a "chignon," and it normally fades away within 48 hours.

- A bruise on a baby's head is called "cephalohematoma." It affects 1 to 12 out of every 100 babies delivered with a ventouse. There's no cause for concern, and the bruise goes away with time.

- Marks on a baby's face from forceps. They disappear within a day or two.

- One in ten babies born via assisted delivery experience minor cuts on their face or scalp; they heal fast.

- Jaundice, which causes your baby's skin and eyes to turn yellow, should subside in a few days.

After an assisted delivery, you may stay in the hospital a little longer, but your recuperation time will be about the same as it would be for a natural birth. It takes around six weeks, but it can take longer if you're recovering from third- or fourth-degree tears. After about a month, the stitches dissolve. You should be able to control any lingering pain with over-the-counter drugs. Consult your healthcare practitioner if the pain is more serious.

The Placenta

Delivery after vaginal birth

Your uterus will continue to contract after the baby is born, so the placenta can advance. These contractions lack the intensity of labor contractions.

Sometimes you may be advised to push harder or have pressure applied to your tummy to get it out. Normally, it's out within 5 minutes, but some people may need more time.

Once you've given birth, you could be so preoccupied with meeting your baby that you don't even feel the placenta delivery. But, some women have reported having seen a second rush of blood that's typically followed by the placenta.

The umbilical cord is connected to the placenta. It doesn't hurt when it's severed because it doesn't have any nerves.

Delivery after cesarean

Your doctor will manually remove the placenta from your uterus during a cesarean delivery before stitching up the incisions.

The fundus (the top portion of your uterus) is then likely to be massaged after birth to help it contract and begin to shrink. They might prescribe medicine, like pitocin, to make your uterus contract if it's unable to do so naturally.

Your placenta will then be carefully checked to ensure it's fully intact after delivery. If it's found to have portions missing, your doctor can advise a uterine ultrasound to confirm. Excessive bleeding after delivery can be a sign that some placenta remains in the uterus. This is called "retained placenta."

Retained Placenta

The following factors could prevent the placenta from delivering fully:

- The cervix closes, leaving a very small gap through which the placenta can't pass.

- The placenta is too firmly fused to the uterine wall.

- During delivery, a piece of the placenta broke off and stayed behind.

The uterus must contract after delivery, so retaining the placenta is a serious risk. Once the uterus is tightened, the blood vessels inside it can stop bleeding. So having portions of the placenta left inside may cause bleeding or infection.

Your doctor will advise surgical removal as soon as possible.

In rare cases, the placenta is so closely bound to the uterus that the only way to remove it is a full hysterectomy.

If you have any of the following, you're at risk of having a retained placenta, for example:

- Prior instances of placenta retention.

- Prior to cesarean delivery.

- Having had uterine fibroids.

Should you be concerned about retaining your placenta, speak with your doctor so they can come up with a strategy to avoid it.

Once the mammoth task of delivering your baby is done, the doctors and nurses have to shift their attention a little bit to make sure your little one is okay. Shortly after giving you a bit of time with baby, they will start running routine tests and monitoring the both of you.

What Is an Apgar Score?

At one and five minutes after birth, babies are given the Apgar test. How well they tolerated labor is measured by the one-minute score. The five-minute score informs the medical professional of the baby's health outside the womb.

In some cases, the test gets carried out ten minutes after delivery.

The Apgar score was first created in 1952 by Virginia Apgar, MD (1909–1974).

A doctor, midwife, or nurse can perform the test. They look at the baby's:

- Heartbeat

- Skin color

- respiratory effort

- Muscle tone

- Reflexes

Each category receives a score of zero, one, or two depending on the baby's condition.

Heart rate

- Babies with no heartbeat receive a score of 0.

- Babies with a heart rate of less than 100 beats per minute receive a score of 1.

- Babies with heart rates over 100 beats per minute receive a score of 2.

Skin color

- If the baby's skin is pale blue, they receive a score of 0.

- If the baby's skin is pink, but their extremities are blue, they receive a score of 1.

- If the baby's skin is pink all over, they receive a score of 2.

Respiratory effort

- If the baby isn't breathing, they receive a score of 0.

- If the baby's breathing is slow and erratic, they receive a score of 1.

- If the baby cries straight after birth, they receive a score of 2.

Muscle tone

- Babies with loose, flaccid muscles receive a score of 0.

- Babies with a bit of muscle tone receive a score of 1.

- Babies that make vigorous movements receive a score of 2.

Reflexes

- If the baby doesn't respond to mild stimulation, they receive a score of 0.

- If the baby grimaces, they receive a score of 1.

- If the baby grimaces, coughs, sneezes, or cries loudly, they receive a score of 2.

Newborn Screening Tests

Your baby will undergo newborn screening when they are one to two days old. At birth, they are screened for dangerous but uncommon and usually treatable medical conditions. It involves tests for the heart, hearing, and blood.

Some babies are born with health conditions and don't show any signs, so screening can help find the ailment early so it can be treated. Early intervention is crucial since it could protect your baby from more serious health issues.

In the United States, newborn screening is provided for every baby. Every year, almost 4 million newborns are screened.

How's It Done?

1. **Hearing test**

    Used to test for hearing loss. Babies wear tiny headphones, and a sophisticated computer is used to monitor how they react to sound.

2. **Heart screening**

    Used to check for a class of heart diseases known as critical congenital heart defects (also called "critical CHDs" or "CCHDs"). It makes use of a quick test known as pulse oximetry. Using a pulse oximeter device and sensors applied to your baby's skin, pulse oximetry measures the amount of oxygen in your baby's blood.

3. **Blood test**

    The blood test is administered to look for uncommon but dangerous medical disorders. Your baby's heel is pricked by a medical professional to obtain a few droplets of blood. They draw the blood onto a piece of paper and send it to a laboratory for analysis. By the time baby is five to seven days old, the results are ready. Ask your baby's doctor or the hospital staff for further information about the timelines for shipping blood samples to the lab and receiving test results back.

What if the Results Aren't Normal?

Most of these tests come back normal. If your baby's results are abnormal, they may just require additional testing. A diagnostic test is the next step to determine whether the baby has a health issue. Further testing is not required if the diagnostic test findings are normal. Your provider can advise you on what to do for your baby if the results are not normal.

One of the most common conditions we see in newborn babies is:

Jaundice

Bilirubin accumulation in the blood is the primary cause of jaundice. The breakdown of red blood cells results in the production of the yellow substance bilirubin.

Jaundice is common among newborns because they have a large amount of red blood cells that are constantly being broken down and replenished. Also, because a newborn baby's liver is still developing, it is less efficient at clearing bilirubin from the blood. The liver becomes more adept at processing bilirubin by the time they are about 2 weeks old, so jaundice resolves by this time without any negative effects on baby.

Jaundice can be hard to see on darker skin tones, so in those cases, you'd look at the palms and the soles of the feet.

Other signs of neonatal jaundice:

- Urine that is dark yellow (newborn babies' pee should be colorless).

- Light-colored poop (it should be yellow or orange)

These symptoms often manifest two days after birth and tend to subside on their own by the time the infant is about two weeks old.

Chapter 12: Postpartum

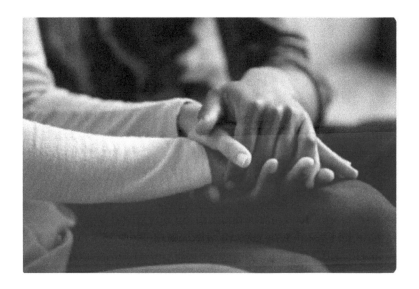

Emotions After Delivery

After you give birth, you go through a range of emotions that words can't describe. Your baby's here, your body still sort of feels pregnant, and your hormones are all over the place. It takes time for everything to balance out and go back to normal, so sometimes, as your body is adjusting, you can experience feelings of dread and anxiety.

In some cases, it manifests as full-on depression.

A lot of new moms go through the *baby blues*, which include unbalanced moods, bouts of crying throughout the day, anxiety, and trouble sleeping. It usually starts a couple of days after delivery and can last up to two weeks. Anything longer than that is most likely postpartum depression.

Postpartum depression is a more severe and pervasive type of depression that new moms endure. If it starts during pregnancy and persists after childbirth, it's called "peripartum depression." In very rare cases, some moms develop postpartum psychosis, which is a severe mood illness.

Postpartum depression is neither a weakness nor a deficiency in a person's character. A lot of the time, it's just a side effect of childbirth. Treating it as soon as possible will help you control your symptoms and strengthen your relationship with your baby.

Signs to Look Out For: Baby Blues

- Anxiety

- Weepiness

- Despair

- Moodiness

- Mood swings

- Trouble concentrating

- Increase or decrease in appetite

- Insomnia

Signs to Look Out For: Postpartum Depression

Postpartum depression can start off feeling like the baby blues, but the symptoms are more severe and persistent. So much so that they could eventually make it difficult for you to take care of your child and do other everyday tasks. Symptoms typically start to appear within the first few weeks of you being a mom, but they can start sooner—during pregnancy—or later—up to a year after delivery.

Symptoms include:

- All the symptoms mentioned above

- Excessive crying

- Withdrawing from those around you

- Having a hard time bonding with your baby

- Sleeping too often

- Fatigue

- Loss of interest and enjoyment in previously enjoyable activities

- Feelings of inadequacy

- Thoughts of self-harm and harming your baby

- Recurring suicidal thoughts

Signs to Look Out For: Postpartum Psychosis

Postpartum psychosis often appears within the first week following delivery. The symptoms are severe. Symptoms include:

- Paranoia

- Being very energized and unhappy

- Trouble sleeping

- Delusions and hallucination

- Feelings of obsession around your baby

- Feeling lost and confused

- Attempting to hurt yourself or your child

Postpartum psychosis needs to be treated right away because it might cause life-threatening ideas or actions.

Can My Partner Have Postpartum Depression?

According to studies, new dads can also experience postpartum depression. They can exhibit symptoms that mimic those of mothers with postpartum depression. They might experience changes in their regular eating and sleeping schedules, or they can feel depressed, exhausted, overwhelmed, or anxious.

The fathers who are most susceptible to postpartum depression are those who are young, have a history of depression, have issues in their relationship, or are financially strapped. PPD in your partner can have the same detrimental effects on your relationship and the development of your child as it would if you had it.

When to Seek Help

It sounds unrealistic, but it can be very hard to even realize, let alone acknowledge, that you've got the baby blues or PPD. If you show any signs, make an appointment with your obstetrician, gynecologist, or primary care physician. Get help as quickly as you can if you exhibit symptoms that point to postpartum psychosis.

Postpartum Body

Your hormones change during pregnancy to promote the development of your unborn child and get your body ready for labor. Once you give birth, they work to help your body recover, foster a bond with your newborn, and help you breastfeed.

The initial hormonal changes following delivery are:

- A decrease in estrogen and progesterone.

- The bonding hormone, oxytocin, increases and plays a part in the powerful maternal instinct you'll experience.

- To signal the production of milk, prolactin levels rise.

Your First Postpartum Period

The restarting of your period following delivery depends on a number of factors. The biggest being whether you've decided to exclusively nurse your baby.

Those who choose not to breastfeed usually get their period between four weeks and three months after giving birth, which is a lot sooner than those who do. Some breastfeeding moms get their period during that time period too, but most don't until they've started to wean or have completely stopped breastfeeding.

Postpartum Hair Loss

In the six months following childbirth, your hair may start to shed or even come out in clumps.

Most people lose around 100 hairs daily, but they don't fall out all at once, so you don't notice. When you're pregnant, your hormones prevent your hair from falling out, making it appear thicker.

Once you've delivered and your hormone levels return to normal, the hair you retained in pregnancy starts to fall out, so it can seem like you're losing hair.

Don't panic though, because you're not losing anything; just going back to normal. If you're breastfeeding, you may retain a bit of that hair, until such time as you decide to wean.

In about a year, everything should have stabilized, and you should start to see your hair going back to the way it was pre-pregnancy.

How You Can Deal With It

- **Get the proper nutrients**: Eat clean and continue taking your prenatal vitamins.

- **Be gentle with your hair**: Use a good conditioner, a wide-toothed comb, and only shampoo when absolutely necessary. This will help reduce tangling.

- **Choose the appropriate accessories**: Instead of using elastic bands to hold hair up, use scrunchies or barrettes, and avoid pulling hair into tight ponytails.

- **Use less heat**: Try to avoid using flat irons, curling irons, and blow dryers.

- **Less chemical treatments**: Postpone getting your hair straightened, permed, or highlighted until the shedding stops.

Postpartum Preeclampsia

Postpartum Preeclampsia is a dangerous disorder associated with high blood pressure. Any new mom who has just had a baby is susceptible. It's the same as preeclampsia in pregnancy but doesn't harm the baby.

Risks include:

- Death

- Organ failure

- Stroke

- Seizures

Warning signs:
- Abdominal pain (upper right quadrant)

- Swelling of the face and hands

- Nausea or vomiting

- Terrible headache

- Seeing spots (or other changes in vision)

- Respiratory issues or shortness of breath

Precautionary measures:
- Rely on your instincts

- Monitor your blood pressure

- Look out for warning signs and tell your doctor

- Determine whether a one-week follow-up appointment is required.

- Don't miss any follow-up appointments

Settling to Breastfeeding

For roughly the first month, new babies should be breastfed 8–12 times each day. Breastmilk is very easily digestible, so babies feel hungry all the time. Regular feedings in the first few weeks also help to promote your milk supply.

By the second month, baby will probably only be nursing seven to nine times a day.

Breastfeeding should be an on-demand thing in the first few weeks. That's roughly every 1.5 to 3 hours. The older babies get, the less they nurse. They also start to develop a more regular eating pattern. For some, it's every 90 minutes, while others wait two to three hours between feeds.

The span of time between feeds should never exceed four hours, even at night.

How do I measure the time between feeds?

The best way to measure the intervals between feeds is to count from the time baby starts feeding as opposed to when they finish. So if baby's first feed was at 5 a.m., and the subsequent feedings began at 7 a.m. and 9 a.m., respectively, you can safely say they're feeding every two hours.

In the beginning, it can definitely feel like all you're doing is nursing, but as the weeks pass, the time between feeds will start to increase.

How long should my baby nurse?

In the beginning, babies can take up to 20 minutes to nurse on both breasts. As they get older and become used to feeding, this may decrease and become five to ten minutes on each side.

The length of time your baby feeds depends on your baby's needs and whether or not:

- Your breast milk has come in (usually two to five days after birth).

- Your let-down reflex happens immediately into a feed. Let-down reflex is the thing that allows milk to flow from the nipple.

- Your flow is fast.

- Baby has a strong latch and can fit as much of your areola as possible in their mouth.

- Baby starts swallowing right away.

- Baby is sleepy or preoccupied.

When to alternate

Try your best to give each breast an equal amount of time to nurse throughout the day by switching while feeding. This helps maintain your milk production in both breasts and helps you avoid uncomfortable engorgement.

If you start with your left breast at a particular feeding time, then try to start with the right one the next time. If you know you struggle to remember things like this, you can do something to help yourself remember. Like putting a ribbon or safety pin on the side of the breast you started the feed with. If you've got the time and energy, you can use a notebook or an app to keep track.

Some babies do favor one breast over the other, so if you can't alternate during a feed, you can just switch between breasts at every feed. Don't put too much pressure on yourself to switch in the middle of a feed. Do what's comfortable for you and baby.

How often to burp

Try burping before switching. Sometimes just the motion of switching can be enough to make a baby burp.

Some babies need a lot of burping, some need less. It depends on the baby, and it can be a different story at every feed.

Burping frequently could help if your baby spits up a lot. Spitting up is normal, but a baby shouldn't vomit after eating. If you notice your baby spitting up all or most of a feed, you may need to seek medical care.

When should I stop?

Do whatever works best for you and your baby. The recommendation is exclusively for 4 to 6 months before introducing solids. Breastfeeding can continue with solids for up to a year or longer as a matter of choice. Try and do it for as long as you can because there are so many benefits for both you and baby.

According to studies, it can reduce a baby's risk of developing diarrhea, ear infections, and bacterial meningitis, or at least minimize the severity of the symptoms. Children who breastfeed are also less susceptible to asthma, diabetes, obesity, and SIDS.

Breastfeeding reduces uterine size and burns calories for mothers. In fact, moms who do might regain their pre-pregnancy weight and shape faster. Moreover, it lowers a woman's risk of developing:

- breast cancer

- hypertension

- heart disease and diabetes

It also could shield moms from ovarian and uterine cancer.

Breastfeeding Twins: Positions and Tips

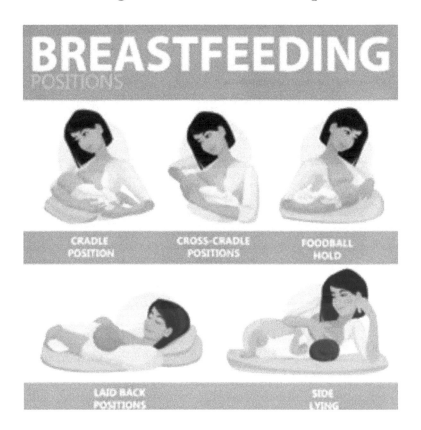

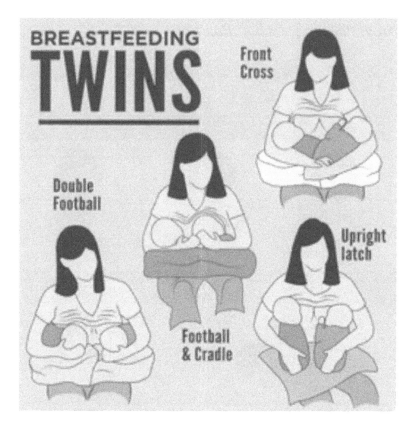

Conceptualizing how to breastfeed twins is quite daunting. You might wrestle with the idea of feeding them one-at-a-time vs at the same time. You should do your best to have them on the same schedule and nursing at the same time. Keeping one hungry baby fed every couple of hours is a big undertaking; imagine that with two.

Here are some tips for nursing twins simultaneously:

Positioning

Nursing while sitting up can be hard, especially when it's nighttime feeding, but that's the safest and most efficient way to get both babies fed.

Find your position by process of elimination. Try out various positions until you find the most effective and pleasant one (Fierro, 2020):

- **Double or cross cradle hold**: A combination of the football and cradle holds. Both babies' torsos and legs are pointed to the side and in the same direction as they lay across mom. Their heads and upper backs are cradled by mom's hands and arms. One baby's legs are tucked under mom's arm (like in the football hold). And baby number two's head can actually rest on their sibling's body.

- **Criss-cross or front-V Hold**: Mom's hands cradle the babies' bodies from below while their heads rest on her forearms. Their legs are pointed in different directions as their bodies are crossed on Mom's lap.

- **Parallel or Saddle Hold**: Both babies are facing mom's chest while seated upright. Ideal for older babies who can sit.

Twins can breastfeed comfortably on a bed, sofa or large armchair. Choose a space where there's enough room for everyone to spread out comfortably and where you can arrange everything you need so that it's close enough for you to reach. Before you start the feed, make sure you've got everything you'll need close by so you don't have to get up and interrupt the session. Make sure the babies are easy to reach before taking position. Try to alternate the babies so that both have access to each breast.

Breast engorgement

Breast engorgement is painful. It feels like they could pop at any time—it also feels warm, sensitive, heavy, and hard to the touch. Besides being uncomfortable, it can also lead to problems breastfeeding, so if you're able to recognize it early enough, you can get it treated.

A good number of moms experience it in the first few weeks. Hormone levels are changing, and milk production is high, so they swell. It's more than just the milk that makes them swell. Your breasts are on the receiving end of extra blood and fluids for milk production, so they swell and become congested. As time goes on and your body starts to go back to normal, it stops.

Causes

- **A feeding schedule**: The amount of milk a moms' breasts can hold without feeling uncomfortable varies. Moms who don't feed on demand regularly experience engorgement, mastitis, and insufficient milk production because their breasts aren't drained frequently enough.

- **Expressing**: Some moms like to kick their milk production into high gear by expressing and making more milk than their babies require. But if you find yourself going hours without expressing or nursing, your breasts can become engorged.

- **A baby that isn't latching**: You can maintain production and prevent clogged ducts or mastitis by routinely expressing milk until your baby is able to nurse comfortably.

- **Weaning too quickly**: Weaning can't happen all at once. It has to be gradual, so that your breasts can get used to producing less and less milk with time. Try hand- or pump-expressing just enough milk to relieve the feeling of fullness, being sure never to fully empty your breasts.

Treatment

- Try to nurse every 1.5 to 2 hours during the day and every 2–3 hours at night, starting at the same time each time. Try to make sure the first breast is empty before moving on to the second.

- To minimize swelling in between feeds, apply ice for 15 to 20 minutes at a time. You can use ice in any form as long as you're protecting your skin with some sort of cloth.

- Apply moist warmth to your breasts just before feeding for up to two minutes to encourage flow. Try a warm shower, a warm cloth, or submerging your breasts in warm water.

Clogged Ducts

Your breasts host a network of mammary ducts that transport milk from the breast to the nipple. If something like inflammation in the surrounding blood vessels and soft tissues obstructs the duct, milk may back up in them.

When a milk duct becomes blocked or obstructed, breast milk can't flow to the nipple.

It manifests as a red, tender, and an uncomfortable lump in your breast. It's crucial to understand the symptoms and how to treat it at home because it can result in infection.

Other symptoms include:

- Swelling or discomfort around the lump.

- Letdown causes pain.

- The disappearance of a lump after a feed or a pump.

- The disappearance of pain and discomfort after a feed.

Some moms get a blister on the nipple. It's called a "bleb." It's a tiny white dot on the nipple made up of debris from inflammation.

The causes of clogged ducts are the same as the ones for engorgement.

Treatment

The abbreviation BAIT can help you recall some of the best methods for unclogging a blocked duct:

- Breast rest: Avoid overstimulation or overfeed. If you are producing too much, reduce your output.

- Advil: Take 800 milligrams every eight hours for two days.

- Ice: Lay on your back and apply ice for ten minutes at a time every 30 minutes.

- Tylenol: Take 1,000 milligrams of Tylenol every eight hours for two days.

Mastitis (an infection) can develop as a result of not treating a blocked milk duct.

Mastitis

Mastitis symptoms develop fairly quickly. They include:

- Chills and body aches.

- Fever

- Red, swollen, pain-filled breasts

- Severe pain while breastfeeding or pumping

If you experience any symptoms, call your obstetrician right away because it needs to be treated with antibiotics.

Bottle-Feeding

How to Prepare Utensils

Everything you need for a bottle-feed must be sterilized and properly prepared. Poor cleanliness or improper preparation could make a baby gravely ill.

These are the steps to follow:

1. Sanitize your hands.

2. In warm, soapy water, clean the bottles, discs, lids, teats, and tongs.

3. Follow the manufacturer's recommendations while sterilizing. Everything can be sterilized using boiling water, a steam kit, or a chemical sterilizer. The best sterilizer is a steam one. Microwaveable or plug-in sterilizers are good too.

4. Before removing the bottles from the sterilizer with the tongs, wash and dry your hands.

5. After sterilization, do not rinse the utensils.

If your bottles are closed properly after sterilization, they will be clean and ready to use for up to 24 hours.

How to Prepare Formula

You'll need the following:

- a sterile prep area

- a minimum of six bottles, lids, discs, and teats

- formula

- a reliable source of water

- A kettle

- a little teat brush and a bottle brush

Use wide-necked bottles if you have vision problems, as they are easier to work with and fill.

These are the steps to follow:

1. Boil water in a kettle, then leave to cool for no longer than 30 minutes. This is so that the water is at least 150 °F.

2. Clean your prep space thoroughly. Use soap and warm water to wash your hands and a fresh towel to dry them.

3. To determine how much water and powder you need, carefully read the directions on the label of the formula.

4. Pour the stipulated amount of boiled water into a sterilized bottle. Be careful, it's still hot.

5. Add the stipulated number of scoops to the bottle. Too much or too little can make baby ill. Properly reseal the container to keep out moisture and germs.

6. To mix, gently swirl the bottle around until well mixed, or use a sterilized spoon to stir. Avoid shaking the bottle to avoid air bubbles.

7. Set the bottle in a big bowl of cold water if you need to cool it down quickly. Just make sure the cold water doesn't go over the bottle's neck or touch the neck.

8. Pour a tiny bit of milk on the inside of your wrist to make sure it's not hot. It should be lukewarm.

9. Feed baby and dispose of any milk the baby didn't drink in two hours.

10. Wash and rinse the bottle after every feed.

How to Give a Bottle

Sit so that you and baby are comfortable.

Always keep the bottle in your hand and baby in your arms.

Never let your child feed on their own. While feeding, your baby maintains eye contact with you, and this helps with bonding and can give you a bit of time to relax.

Never rest the bottle on or lean it against:

- a regular pillow

- a self-feeding pillow

- any other support structure

Your baby might choke if you do this.

Paced Feeding

Pacing is so important. Your baby will be able to regulate how quickly and how much milk they consume.

The best way for you and baby to get used to bottle-feeding is through paced feeding. It's comfortable for baby, and you can avoid overfeeding.

These are the steps to follow:

1. Hold the bottle horizontally while holding baby in an upright position on your lap.

2. Play around baby's top lip with the teat until they open their mouth.

3. Let baby suckle on the teat.

4. Tilt the bottle ever so slightly so that the teat fills with milk.

5. When baby stops for a break, lower the bottle so there's no milk in the teat.

6. Look to your baby for cues on when to feed and when to pause. Stop when they appear satisfied.

When your baby has had enough, they'll show it, so don't feed them beyond what they're willing to handle.

You can use a cup with handles if your child is older than six months and prefers not to drink from a bottle.

Until baby learns how to feed themself, only pour a small amount of liquid into the cup at a time. This will save you from lots of spillage and waste.

To avoid excessive spitting up or vomiting, keep baby upright for at least 30 minutes after feeding. Use a smaller teat if you are experiencing issues with vomiting. If a teat is too big for your baby, it probably has a much faster flow and that may be triggering your baby's gag reflex.

Bonding With Your Baby

The universal idea of mothers bonding with their babies, is that they are immediately connected to their babies the second they're born. That's true for some, and not for others.

You carried your baby, so you've loved them from the beginning, that's a given. But the truth is that once the baby's out, they're essentially a stranger. It's normal for you to need some time to get to know them.

Many new parents require a bit of time to connect. When you bond with your baby, you start to feel an unwavering love for them. It's something that develops gradually, sometimes over the course of a year. So it's perfectly okay if you don't experience these intense feelings in the first few days or weeks following delivery.

There are things you can do to foster a close relationship with your baby, but there are also things that can impede the bonding process. It will eventually happen with time and with constant, close contact with your baby.

Why is it important?

Bonding is essential for development.

Your baby will believe the world is a safe place to play, learn, and explore when they get what they need from you. It could be as small as a smile, touch, or snuggle. These things establish the framework for your child's growth and welfare throughout childhood.

The act of bonding promotes your baby's physical and mental development. Frequent human interaction causes the baby's brain to release hormones. These hormones promote brain development. And, as your baby's brain develops, memory, cognition, and language develop too.

How to bond with your baby

Try the following:

- Speak to your baby in calming, reassuring tones. You could talk about the weather, or tell tales. Your baby will learn to recognize the sound of your voice and have a good foundation on which to learn language as they get older.

- Sing. Your baby will probably enjoy the rhythm and tones of songs and music.

- Look your baby in the eye when you talk and sing. Express yourself with your face too; that way, your baby will learn the relationship between words and feelings.

- Touch and cuddle your baby often. They can sense even the slightest touch. Gently stroke your baby when you're doing mundane things like changing a diaper or giving a bath.

- Always respond when your baby cries. Even if you haven't the slightest clue why they're crying, your responsiveness indicates to them that you'll always be there for them.

- Hold your baby close. Set some time aside to rock or cuddle your baby skin-to-skin.

- Make your baby feel secure physically. When holding your child, support their head and neck well. You can also swaddle them to mimic the safe environment of the womb.

Even after taking these steps, you might not feel the bond with your child that you believe you should, but there's no need to feel bad or embarrassed. The bond will develop the more time you spend together. More so if you've got support and time for self-care.

Here are some things to look out for that might slow the process of you bonding with your baby:

- The baby blues

- Postpartum depression

- A lack of support and time for self-care

Baby's First Bath

For a lot of parents, bath time is their favorite time to spend with their new babies. It's a great opportunity to connect without any interruptions. But these days, there's a lot of debate (mostly online) about how and when to bathe your newborn. Something that was a standard practice for centuries is now a source of uncertainty and even fear.

Most hospitals have typically washed babies within the first hour of their birth, but that's changing.

The World Health Organization advises waiting at least 24 hours after birth—or at least 6 hours if a full day is impractical for cultural reasons—before giving a newborn its first bath.

Reasons why it's recommended to delay the first bath include:

Breastfeeding and bonding: Premature bathing of the infant can interfere with early breastfeeding, skin-to-skin contact, and bonding. One study found that delaying the baby's initial bath by 12 hours led to a 166% increase in nursing success compared to babies who were bathed right away.

Dry skin: The vernix is a white waxy substance that covers babies' skin prior to birth. It's like a natural moisturizer and may have antibacterial properties. It should be left on the skin for a while to prevent the drying out of their sensitive skin. Preemies would greatly benefit from this because of how easily their skin can be damaged.

Blood sugar levels and body temperature: Babies who get bathed immediately could be more susceptible to hypothermia. Also, for some babies, that first bath can feel slightly stressful, which can increase their risk of experiencing a decrease in blood sugar (hypoglycemia).

Babies don't require baths every day because they don't perspire or become unclean enough to need them.

For the first year, three baths a week are enough. Anything more than that can cause your baby's skin to become dry.

Stick to sponge baths for the first couple of weeks or until the cord falls off.

Safety tips for a sponge bath:

- Ensure you've got everything ready before you start.

- Place baby on a flat surface that's comfortable for them, and convenient for you.

- Wash baby's face first.

- Keep baby warm.

You can start immersing your baby in water once the belly button area is healed. It's best to be gentle and quick with his first few baths. If baby seems at all uncomfortable, you can go back to giving sponge baths for a week or so, then try a normal bath again. Your baby will let you know when they're ready to make the switch.

Safety tips for a regular bath:

- Use a baby bath or sink.

- Don't use bath seats.

- Use touch supervision.

- Never leave a baby alone in the bath, even for an instant.

- Check the water temperature.

- Keep baby warm.

- Use soap sparingly as it dries the skin.

- Clean gently.

- Have fun.

- Get out, dry off, and moisturize.

Once you've got the fundamentals down, bath time becomes so easy. Just make sure baby is safe and comfortable, and don't forget to enjoy every moment.

Looking After the Cord

It can take up to three weeks for the umbilical cord stump to dry out and fall off. Here's how you can gently treat the belly button area in the interim:

- **Keep it dry**: Once upon a time, parents were told to swab the stump with rubbing alcohol following each diaper change. It's been discovered that this may destroy bacteria that dries the cord so it can fall off. It's best to just let it breathe. To avoid suffocating it, keep the front of your baby's diaper folded down.

- **Only do sponge baths**: Although getting the stump wet is harmless, sponge baths make it easier to keep it dry.

- **Let it fall off naturally**: Avoid the urge to remove the stump yourself.

Things to lookout for:

It's common to notice a little blood close to the stump as it heals. The cord stump may bleed a little when it comes off, similar to a scab.

But, if the umbilical area oozes pus, the surrounding skin turns red and inflamed, or the area forms a pink, moist bump, call your baby's healthcare practitioner. These might be indicators of an infection in the umbilical cord. To prevent the illness from spreading, quick treatment is required.

Moreover, if the stump hasn't detached after three weeks, consult your baby's doctor. This could be a symptom of a deeper issue, like an infection or immune system dysfunction.

Six Weeks Postpartum

Sex After Delivery

A lot of women swear off sex once they've given birth, but it's just talk. It's bound to happen at some point. Chances are you won't be in the mood, and it may be a bit uncomfortable at first, but here's all you need to know:

How Soon After Delivery Can I Do It?

The medically approved time frame, regardless of delivery method, is four to six weeks. If you're going to experience any post-birth complications, it's likely to happen in the first two weeks following delivery. So waiting will allow your body more time to recover.

You may also have a reduced sex drive, exhaustion, vaginal dryness, pain, postpartum discharge, and vaginal tears. You might have to wait longer if your vaginal tear needs surgical repair.

Will It Hurt and What Can I Do?

Your vagina may become dry and sore due to hormonal changes, especially if you breastfeed. If you are recovering from an episiotomy or perineal tears, you could feel some discomfort during sex as well.

To make it more comfortable:

- **Pain management**: Try to prepare by taking pain-relieving measures like emptying your bladder, having a warm bath, or taking an over-the-counter (OTC) painkiller. Use ice wrapped in a cloth towel on the area if you feel a burning sensation.

- **Employ lubricant**: If you feel vaginal dryness.

- **Experiment**: Talk about alternatives to penetrative sex, like reciprocal masturbation, massages, and oral sex. Be honest about what feels good and what doesn't.

- **Set aside time**: Schedule sex if you need to. Preferably when you're not too tired or nervous.

What Can I Do if I'm Just Not Interested?

When adjusting to life after delivery, there is more to intimacy than just sex. Be open with your spouse. If you're not feeling sexy or if you're worried that it will hurt, communicate that. Keep up your intimacy in other ways until you're ready to engage in sex. Even if it's just a few minutes when you get a break, or after the baby goes to sleep, spend time alone together. Find different ways to show your love.

If you're still having trouble, keep an eye out for postpartum depression's telltale signs and symptoms. Contact your doctor if you suspect postpartum depression. Early intervention means early healing.

Always remember that maintaining good health and making time for self-care might help you keep the passion alive.

What Are the Positives?

Quickies are here to save the day: Fun tidbit about sex after birth: It doesn't have to last for hours on end. Have your spouse stimulate you, and then you do everything in your power to maintain your interest in the present. To stay present, concentrate on the feeling of what's being done to you and what you're doing in return.

Sex doesn't only have to happen at night: Weekends, during baby's nap, is the ideal time to connect. It can relieve some of the pressure you might feel at night and become something to look forward to.

It could get better after birth: It sounds strange, but many moms find that they enjoy sex more now than they did before becoming parents. Delivering a baby exposes us to a variety of feelings, and as a result, our bodies—particularly our genitalia—become more sensitive, enhancing our capacity for pleasure.

Our internal organs can also be precisely repositioned during childbirth, increasing their receptivity to stimulation.

Your sex drive will eventually come back: You'll want to have sex again after giving birth, the same way you'll want to sleep again, go on outings, and even give birth again. Give yourself time to heal and get used to your new lifestyle.

Contrary to popular belief, having more children does not mean having less sex. You will eventually come to the realization that life with kids will always be hectic, but you simply have to soldier on and have fun whenever and wherever you can.

Common Partnership Issues After Baby and How to Solve Them

The transition from coupledom to parenthood is thrilling, exhilarating, and amazing. It's also taxing, frustrating, and worrying—a combination that could be harmful to the romantic bond that originally led to you becoming parents.

Sustaining a marriage after having a child requires a lot of time and effort, which is ironic because those are probably the two things you don't have. Making efforts to maintain your relationship pays off in the long run. You'll have more time to spend appreciating one another because you won't spend much time feeling resentful of one another.

Here's why it's so hard, and how you can make things go more smoothly:

- **Chores**: Before having a baby, it was easier to get chores done. But the chores don't disappear once baby's home. If chores pile up, it can lead to frustration on both sides. So the best thing to do is have a visual aid in place that states which chores need to be done and by whom. Alternate if you need to, and always be clear about what you need. Nobody can read your mind, so be direct. Make it a standard practice to thank your partner after they finish a task. They might be more responsive to requests in the future if you express gratitude. Niceties also foster a more healthy environment.

- **Difference of opinion**: Not many people have parenting plans in place, and the conversations about how things should be done don't happen as often as you'd think. It's usually once the baby arrives that parents start to notice how different their opinions on raising babies are. If parent A chooses to do things their way, they should be willing to deal with whatever happens as a result of the method they employ. For instance, the parent who lets the baby take a nap too close to bedtime should be willing to stay up with the baby when they won't sleep. Compromises should be made on issues like feeding and sleep training. There is enough information out there to allow parents to come to an agreement.

- **Less quality time**: Before baby, there was probably a nice balance between your personal lives and your life as a couple. After baby, you probably spend more time together, but it's not in a way you're used to. You're together all the time, but because it's not quality time, there becomes a disconnect. The solution is to carve out alone time for yourselves as individuals, time to enjoy each other's company as a couple, and family time. Balance is key.

- **No alone time**: A baby is a round-the-clock commitment, so it's no wonder you don't get time to yourself. The first three months are likely to be all about baby, but after that, you should start considering ways to pop out and do something for yourself.

- **Potentially overbearing family**: Grandparents love grandchildren, aunts, and uncles love niblings. It's good for your baby to be surrounded by and showered with love, but you have to put boundaries in place before extended family overwhelms you. Try and think of the rules you'd like to enforce for your family before you give birth. Communicate them, so that everybody's on the same page and nobody gets hurt.

- **Money worries**: Money is a big deal. It's a contributing factor to the breakdown of a lot of relationships. If you feel stressed about money, you're not going to take it out on your baby, you'll take it out on dad and vice versa. The solution to this is preemptive planning, a lot of talking, and a lot of compromising.

Your First Checkup: What to Expect

A postpartum checkup is a medical exam you have soon after giving birth to make sure you're healing properly. Even if you feel well, you should go. Postpartum care is crucial because new mothers run the risk of developing serious, even fatal health issues in the days and weeks following delivery. Postpartum care reduces the number of new moms who suffer from health issues that could prove fatal.

What's a Postpartum Care Plan?

Together with your healthcare practitioner, you can create a postpartum care plan. It makes it easier to get ready for your postpartum medical treatment. Don't wait to develop your plan until after you deliver. Set it up while you're still pregnant.

Chat with your provider about:

- Their contact details.

- Your postpartum checkups.

- Your reproductive plan and birth control.

- Health issues or post-pregnancy complications that need treatment.

- The normal emotional and physical changes following pregnancy.

- PPD and other mental health issues following pregnancy.

- Feeding baby.

What Happens at a Checkup?

Your healthcare professional checks to make sure you're recuperating after delivery and adjusting to life as a mom. You can expect a full physical that includes:

- Blood pressure, weight, breasts, and belly check
- A pelvic exam
- Checks on any health conditions you had during pregnancy, i.e., diabetes and hypertension
- Check to see if your immunizations are up to date.
- Birth control.

There will also be conversations about any problems you faced while pregnant and your feelings about being a mother.

Baby's First Checkup: What to Expect

Your baby's first checkup will actually be by a pediatrician at the hospital right after the birth. The doctor will perform a physical exam of baby's overall health, assess their reflexes, and offer advice if there are any issues with weight or feeding.

Sometimes, the doctor might need to see your baby a few times a day for the first couple of days in the hospital. This would only happen if your baby has jaundice, or issues with weight or feeding.

The subsequent checkup will normally take place at your preferred clinic three to five days after delivery. Your baby's first week on earth is really important to their health. They are completely new to the world and are learning how to live, and adapt to new surroundings. Everything's new to you too, so doctors want you to know they're there for you.

How Far in Advance Should I Book the Checkup?

How to pick your baby's first doctor? The decision is ultimately up to you, but here's what to take into account:

- Choose a clinic close to home.
- Find a doctor you connect with by reading up on them online.
- Find a practice that lets you easily access baby's medical and immunization records online.
- Choose a medical professional who is well-trained and experienced. Board certification is something you can seek out.

What Happens at the Checkup?

Before the checkup, some clinics require you to fill out online documents pertaining to your baby's health and development and how you're adjusting to motherhood.

Once you arrive, a nurse will gather any additional paperwork you have completed and ask you a few routine questions. They'll also measure your baby's head circumference, length, and weight.

The doctor will then come in and review the growth chart with you to make sure your baby is gaining weight and developing normally. They will also ask about baby's feeding schedule, sleeping habits, and bowel movement.

Finally, the doctor will perform a thorough head-to-toe check to assess baby's general health and look for signs of abnormalities or developmental delays. They'll perform:

- A head check

- A hip check

- A reflex check

- An umbilical cord check

There will be a time in your appointment for you to speak with the doctor and ask any questions. Some clinics have a nurse line that you can call whenever a question comes up or if you feel like you need some guidance.

What Should I Take With Me?

As a new parent, it's natural to feel stressed out, especially when you're sleep deprived. Hence, getting ready for the baby's medical appointment beforehand is a smart method to maintain composure and efficiency.

Here are a few items to bring:

- A bottle

- A blanket

- An extra outfit

- Your insurance card

- Paperwork from the hospital if you have any

- A feeding journal if you keep one

- Diapers and wipes

Conclusion

Dear First-Time Mother,

I want to take a moment to commend you on your incredible journey through pregnancy. The moment you learned you were expecting, your journey of joy, excitement, and anticipation began. And through it all, despite the difficulties and uncertainty of bringing new life into the world, you have exhibited incredible courage, tenacity, and grace.

You have dealt with morning sickness, exhaustion, and a plethora of other physical side effects associated with conceiving a child. You have given your body proper care, fed your child, and made countless other sacrifices. You have balanced the emotional ups and downs that pregnancy can bring while managing your job, household duties, and the never-ending stream of doctor's appointments and testing.

You have shown your unwavering love and dedication to your unborn child throughout it all. You have built a relationship with your infant that will last a lifetime by talking, reading, and singing to them. For the sake of your child's health and welfare, you have made several sacrifices and set aside your own demands.

You could have started this journey as a first time mother feeling unsure and unprepared. To finish this chapter, keep in mind that you have grown into a strong and capable caretaker, equipped with the force of unwavering love and a fresh appreciation for the wondrous experience of motherhood.

I want to remind you that you are a true warrior and an inspiration to everyone you know as you get ready for the next stage of your adventure. You will remain led by your fortitude, tenacity, and love in the coming years. As you continue on your path, please know that you have our love and support as you reach this incredible milestone.

Sincerely yours, Elizabeth Benson

If you have enjoyed this book, please leave a helpful review on Amazon.

Glossary

Albumin: A protein that may show up in your urine during pregnancy. It might be a symptom of preeclampsia or another illness. At your prenatal visits, your midwife will examine your urine for albumin.

Antenatal: It pertains to the entire pregnancy, from conception to delivery, and literally means "before birth."

Birth canal: The pathway that a baby passes through during delivery. It's made up of the cervix, vagina, and vulva.

Catheter: A flexible, thin tube made of plastic that can be used for a variety of therapeutic or diagnostic operations. Catheters can be used for drainage, such as from a surgical site or the bladder, as well as for the injection of fluids or medications into specific bodily parts.

Colostrum: The milk that your breasts produce around the end of your pregnancy and in the early days following the birth of your child. It is highly concentrated and packed with antibodies to guard your infant from infections. Colostrum seems rich and creamy and can occasionally be quite golden in color.

Cot death: The unexpected passing away of a seemingly healthy infant in their sleep. Also known as SIDS.

Down's syndrome: A genetic disorder characterized by an excessive number of chromosomes. People who have Down's syndrome are more likely to experience some health issues and have some degree of learning difficulty. Their facial features and physical development are also impacted.

Dystocia: A labor that stagnates. Shoulder dystocia is when a baby's shoulders become stuck after the head has been delivered; labor dystocia is when contractions do not strengthen and cervical change stops.

Embryo: Refers to the growing baby during the first eight weeks of pregnancy.

Fetus: Refers to the growing baby from eight weeks onwards.

Fundus: The upper part of the womb.

Gingivitis: Red, sensitive, and bleeding gums that can progress into periodontitis, if neglected.

Hemoglobin: Red blood cells contain hemoglobin, which transports oxygen from the lungs to every area of the body. Because they create more blood during pregnancy, pregnant women need to produce more hemoglobin. Insufficient production can cause anemia, which will make you feel extremely exhausted. During prenatal visits, your hemoglobin levels are checked.

Hypotension: Low blood pressure. While in childbirth, some women who receive an epidural experience hypotension.

Hypoxia: When the mother's blood pressure is too low, or the cord is compressed, the baby does not receive enough oxygen.

Lanugo: Fine, soft hair that covers baby at around 22 weeks. At full gestation, the lanugo fades, but it could still be there on premature babies.

Meconium: Your baby's first stools, or bowel movements. Meconium is made up of mucus and bile that babies consumed when they were in the uterus. It has a tar-like consistency, is green or black in color, and is odorless.

Neonatal care: The treatment provided to preterm or ill newborns. It occurs in a neonatal unit, which is especially created and furnished to take care of them.

Oedema: Swelling, most frequently of the hands and feet. Although it is typically nothing to worry about, if your high blood pressure suddenly worsens, it may indicate preeclampsia.

Perinatal: The period just before and following a birth.

Pica: The urge some pregnant women have to eat things like dirt, chalk, or clay. It is believed to be related to anemia caused by iron deficiency.

Postnatal: The window of time from the moment a baby is born until they are roughly six weeks old.

Precipitous birth: One that occurs very quickly, usually in less than three hours.

Rubella: A virus that, if contracted by the mother in the first few weeks of pregnancy, can have a significant impact on unborn children. Since the majority of women have received their rubella vaccinations, they are not in danger. If you are considering becoming pregnant and doubt your immunity to rubella, request a blood test from your doctor.

Steroids: Synthetic hormones that could be administered to a pregnant woman experiencing preterm labor in an effort to hasten the fetus's lung development.

Zygote: The fertilized egg just prior to its first division and development into an embryo.

References

Abedin, S. (2022, September 11). *Water Birth Information: Benefits and Risks of Water Birth.* WebMD. https://www.webmd.com/baby/water-birth

Advantages of bottle-feeding. (n.d.) BIBS. https://bibsworld.com/blogs/guides/advantages-of-bottle-feeding

Aggarwal, N. (2021, November 18). *Postpartum Checkups: When They Occur and What to Expect.* Thebump. https://www.thebump.com/a/postpartum-checkup

Apgar score. (2016). Medlineplus. https://medlineplus.gov/ency/article/003402.htm

Baby movements in pregnancy. (n.d.). Tommys https://www.tommys.org/pregnancy-information/pregnancy-symptom-checker/baby-fetal-movements

Baby's first doctor appointment. (2021, February 18). HealthPartners Blog. https://www.healthpartners.com/blog/what-to-expect-at-babys-first-doctor-appointment/

Back pain during pregnancy: 7 tips for relief. (2019). Mayo Clinic. https://www.mayoclinic.org/healthy-lifestyle/pregnancy-week-by-week/in-depth/pregnancy/art-20046080

Balonwu, V. (2015, December 1). *Miscarriage Causes And Treatment - Health And Medical Information*. Viviennebalonwu. https://www.viviennebalonwu.com/2015/05/miscarriage-causes-and-treatment.html

Bleeding during pregnancy Causes. (2022, January 20). Mayo Clinic. https://www.mayoclinic.org/symptoms/bleeding-during-pregnancy/basics/causes/sym-20050636#:~:text=Normal%20vaginal%20bleeding%20near%20the

Bonding and attachment: newborns. (2020, November 8). Raising Children Network. https://raisingchildren.net.au/newborns/connecting-communicating/bonding/bonding-newborns#when-bonding-and-attachment-arent-easy-nav-title

Braxton Hicks contractions. (n.d.). HSE.ie. https://www2.hse.ie/conditions/braxton-hicks/#:~:text=Braxton%20Hicks%20contractions%20happen%20when

Breast Milk Is Best. (2021b, December 8). Johns Hopkins Medicine. https://www.hopkinsmedicine.org/health/conditions-and-diseases/breastfeeding-your-baby/breast-milk-is-the-best-milk#:~:text=Compared%20with%20formula%2C%20the%20nutrients

Breastfeeding - Common myths. (2022, May 25). HSE.ie. https://www2.hse.ie/babies-children/breastfeeding/a-good-start/common-myths/

Breastfeeding vs. Formula Feeding Information. (2021, May 24). Mount Sinai Health System. https://www.mountsinai.org/health-library/special-topic/breastfeeding-vs-formula-feeding

C-Section (Cesarean Birth): Procedure & Risks. (2022, August 14). Cleveland Clinic. https://my.clevelandclinic.org/health/treatments/7246-cesarean-birth-c-section

C-Section (Cesarean Section): Procedure, Risks & Recovery. (2022, August 14). Cleveland Clinic. https://my.clevelandclinic.org/health/treatments/7246-cesarean-birth-c-section#recovery-and-outlook

Carlson, J. (2020, February 27). *8 Dangers of Smoking While Pregnant.* Healthline. https://www.healthline.com/health/smoking-and-pregnancy

Causes of second trimester loss. (n.d.). The Miscarriage Association. https://www.miscarriageassociation.org.uk/information/miscarriage/second-trimester-loss-late-miscarriage/causes-of-second-trimester-loss/

Charles, A. (2021, June 14). *10 Foods and Drinks with Caffeine.* Healthline. https://www.healthline.com/nutrition/foods-with-caffeine

Choosing your birth partners | Labour & birth articles & support (2022, August 18). National Childbirth Trust. https://www.nct.org.uk/labour-birth/dads-and-partners/choosing-your-birth-

partners#:~:text=Whoever%20you%20choose%20as%20
20your

Clogged Milk Duct: Causes, Symptoms & Treatment. (2022, March 10). Cleveland Clinic. https://my.clevelandclinic.org/health/diseases/24239-clogged-milk-duct

Collier, S. (2021, June 25). *How can you manage anxiety during pregnancy?* Harvard Health. https://www.health.harvard.edu/blog/how-can-you-manage-anxiety-during-pregnancy-202106252512

Common Foods to Avoid. (n.d.). Community Care Midwives. https://communitycaremidwives.com/common-foods-to-avoid.html

Cottrell, S. (2022, April 21). *Is It Safe To Take a Bath While Pregnant?* Parents. https://www.parents.com/pregnancy/my-body/is-taking-a-warm-bath-in-the-last-trimester-safe/

Danielsson, K. (2022, December 6). *Find out When It's Time to Call a Doctor If Your Baby Isn't Kicking.* Verywell Family. https://www.verywellfamily.com/what-to-do-if-your-baby-is-not-kicking-2371400

De Bellefonds, C. (2023, February 24). *Are Changes in Fetal Movement and Baby Kicks Normal?* What to Expect. https://www.whattoexpect.com/pregnancy/fetal-development/changes-in-fetal-movement/#worry

Diehl, W. (2018, May 21). *Do I Have Postpartum Depression or Just the Baby Blues?* Right as Rain by UW Medicine. https://rightasrain.uwmedicine.org/mind/mental-health/do-i-have-postpartum-depression-or-just-baby-blues-0

Doctor, M. (2022, March 15). *Postpartum Check Up: All You Need To Know | theAsianparent Philippines.* Ph.theasianparent.com. https://ph.theasianparent.com/all-you-need-to-know-about-postpartum-check-up

Does a Hot Bath Induce Labor? (2021, March 2). WebMD. https://www.webmd.com/baby/does-a-hot-bath-induce-labor

Donaldson-Evans, C. (2005, April 25). *Watch Your Baby's Growth at Week 4.* WhattoExpect. https://www.whattoexpect.com/pregnancy/week-by-week/week-4.aspx

Donaldson-Evans, C. (2021, June 1). *Why Might Your Practitioner Decide to Induce Labor?* What to Expect. https://www.whattoexpect.com/pregnancy/labor-induction/#definition

Donaldson-Evans, C., & Murkoff, H. (2021a, June 24). *Week 20 of Pregnancy.* What to Expect. https://www.whattoexpect.com/pregnancy/week-by-week/week-20.aspx

Donaldson-Evans, C., & Murkoff, H. (2021b, June 24). *Week 32 of Pregnancy.* What to Expect. https://www.whattoexpect.com/pregnancy/week-by-week/week-32.aspx

Donaldson-Evans, C., & Murkoff, H. (2022a, June 24). *16 Weeks Pregnant.* What to Expect.

https://www.whattoexpect.com/pregnancy/week-by-week/week-16.aspx

Donaldson-Evans, C., & Murkoff, H. (2022b, June 24). *Week 8 of Pregnancy*. What to Expect. https://www.whattoexpect.com/pregnancy/week-by-week/week-8.aspx

Donaldson-Evans, C., & Murkoff, H. (2022c, June 24). *Week 12 of Pregnancy*. What to Expect. https://www.whattoexpect.com/pregnancy/week-by-week/week-12.aspx

Donaldson-Evans, C., & Murkoff, H. (2022d, June 24). *Week 24 of Pregnancy*. What to Expect. https://www.whattoexpect.com/pregnancy/week-by-week/week-24.aspx

Donaldson-Evans, C., & Murkoff, H. (2022e, June 24). *Week 28 of Pregnancy*. What to Expect. https://www.whattoexpect.com/pregnancy/week-by-week/week-28.aspx

Donaldson-Evans, C., & Murkoff, H. (2022f, June 24). *Week 36 of Pregnancy*. What to Expect. https://www.whattoexpect.com/pregnancy/week-by-week/week-36.aspx

Drug use and pregnancy. (2019, April 1). Stanford Medicine. https://www.stanfordchildrens.org/en/topic/default?id=illegal-drug-use-and-pregnancy-85-P01208

Dunkin, M. A. (2022, August 8). *Childbirth Classes: Lamaze, Bradley, Alexander, and Other Types*. WebMD.

https://www.webmd.com/baby/childbirth-class-options

Ectopic pregnancy - Symptoms and causes. (2018, September 8). Mayo Clinic. https://www.mayoclinic.org/diseases-conditions/ectopic-pregnancy/symptoms-causes/syc-20372088

Engorged Breasts - avoiding and treating. (2016, January 28). La Leche League GB. https://www.laleche.org.uk/engorged-breasts-avoiding-and-treating/

Episiotomy why you might need one. (2019, June 19). HSE.ie. https://www2.hse.ie/pregnancy-birth/birth/episiotomy/why-you-might-need-one/

Equipment for bottle-feeding. (2022, September 14). HSE.ie. https://www2.hse.ie/babies-children/bottle-feeding/equipment/

Exercise in Pregnancy. (2020, December 2). NHS https://www.nhs.uk/pregnancy/keeping-well/exercise/

Family Health History and Planning for Pregnancy. (2019). Centers for Disease Control and Prevention. https://www.cdc.gov/genomics/famhistory/famhist_plan_pregnancy.htm

Fierro, P. P. (2020, October 27). *Correctly Positioning Your Twins for Breastfeeding.* Verywell Family. https://www.verywellfamily.com/how-to-breastfeed-twins-together-4114638

Forceps Delivery: What to Expect, Risks & Recovery. (2022, June 12). Cleveland Clinic. https://my.clevelandclinic.org/health/treatments/2326 0-forceps-delivery

Forceps or vacuum delivery. (2020, December 2). NHS https://www.nhs.uk/pregnancy/labour-and-birth/what-happens/forceps-or-vacuum-delivery/

Freeborn, D., Trevino, H. M., & Burd, I. (2022, January 4). *Fetal Monitoring.* Nationwidechildrens.org. https://www.nationwidechildrens.org/conditions/healt h-library/fetal-monitoring

Gestational diabetes - Symptoms and causes. (2017, April 24). Mayo Clinic. https://www.mayoclinic.org/diseases-conditions/gestational-diabetes/symptoms-causes/syc-20355339

Gibran, K. (2018). *On Children by Kahlil Gibran - Poems.* Academy of American Poets. https://poets.org/poem/children-1

Glossary of useful terms. (2009). Hscni.net. https://www.publichealth.hscni.net/

Goodenough, G. (2021, January 18). *The Pros and Cons of Formula Feeding.* Ready, Set, Food! https://readysetfood.com/blogs/community/the-pros-and-cons-of-formula-feeding

Graves, G. (2022, December 4). *A Simple Birth Plan Template for First-Time Parents.* Parents. https://www.parents.com/pregnancy/giving-birth/labor-and-delivery/how-to-write-a-short-simple-birth-plan/

Greenspan, Y. (2016, January 21). *The Importance of Reading While Pregnant.* Literary Hub. https://lithub.com/the-importance-of-reading-while-pregnant/

Group B strep (strep B) and pregnancy. (2020, July 1). Tommy's. https://www.tommys.org/pregnancy-information/pregnancy-complications/group-b-strep-strep-b-and-pregnancy

Group B strep disease - Symptoms and causes. (2019). Mayo Clinic. https://www.mayoclinic.org/diseases-conditions/group-b-strep/symptoms-causes/syc-20351729

Group B Streptococcus (GBS) in pregnancy and newborn babies. (2017, May 1). Royal College of Obstetricians and Gynaecologists. https://www.rcog.org.uk/for-the-public/browse-all-patient-information-leaflets/group-b-streptococcus-gbs-in-pregnancy-and-newborn-babies/

Gurevich, R. (2022, September 16). *Why You Have Mood Swings During Pregnancy and How to Cope.* Verywell Family. https://www.verywellfamily.com/mood-swings-during-pregnancy-4159590

Healthy diet during pregnancy. (2022, June 22). Healthdirect Australia. https://www.pregnancybirthbaby.org.au/healthy-diet-during-pregnancy#balanced-diet

Hecht, A. (2006, December). *Exercise During Pregnancy.* WebMD. https://www.webmd.com/baby/guide/exercise-during-pregnancy

Hepatitis B. (2012, April 25). American Pregnancy Association. https://americanpregnancy.org/womens-health/hepatitis-b/

High Blood Pressure During Pregnancy. (2021, May 6). Centers for Disease Control and Prevention. https://www.cdc.gov/bloodpressure/pregnancy.htm#:~:text=Gestational%20Hypertension&text=It%20is%20typically%20diagnosed%20after

How To Deal With Emotions After Giving Birth. (2017, November 13). Parenthood Times. https://parenthoodtimes.com/emotions-after-giving-birth/

How to give a baby a bottle. (2022, December 14). HSE.ie. https://www2.hse.ie/babies-children/bottle-feeding/how-to-give-baby-bottle/

How your baby is monitored during labour. (2021, November 4). HSE.ie. https://www2.hse.ie/pregnancy-birth/labour/preparing/monitoring/

Howland, G. (2021, October 12). *Mama Natural Birth Course vs. Lamaze Childbirth Classes.* Mama Natural. https://www.mamanatural.com/mama-natural-vs-lamaze-birthing-classes/#:~:text=Lamaze%20focuses%20on%20healthy%20childbirth

I can't stop crying after the birth of my baby. (2019, August 4). National Childbirth Trust. https://www.nct.org.uk/baby-toddler/crying/i-cant-stop-crying-after-birth-my-baby

Iftikhar, N. (2020a, June 27). *How to Know When to Go to the Hospital for Labor.* Healthline. https://www.healthline.com/health/pregnancy/when-to-go-to-the-hospital-for-labor

Iftikhar, N. (2020b, August 31). *Understanding Fetal Position.* Healthline. https://www.healthline.com/health/baby/fetal-position#possible-positions

Inducing labor: When to wait, when to induce. (2022, May 4). Mayo Clinic. https://www.mayoclinic.org/healthy-lifestyle/labor-and-delivery/in-depth/inducing-labor/art-20047557#:~:text=Can%20I%20request%20an%20elective

Kegel Exercises: How to and & Benefits. (2023, January 2). Cleveland Clinic. https://my.clevelandclinic.org/health/articles/14611-kegel-exercises

Larson, J. (2020, April 22). *When to Worry About Fetal Movement: Decreases and Increases.* Healthline. https://www.healthline.com/health/pregnancy/when-to-worry-about-fetal-movement#decreased-movement

Lauretta, A. (2021, August 4). *When To Announce Your Pregnancy.* Forbes Health. https://www.forbes.com/health/family/when-to-announce-pregnancy/

Lessing, D., & Indeed editorial team. (2022, October 1). *55 Inspiring Quotes About Learning (Why They Are Helpful).*

Indeed.com. https://ca.indeed.com/career-advice/career-development/quotes-about-learning

Lukasik, E. (2016, February 3). *Emergency birth: What to do when you can't get to the hospital.* Pregnancy Magazine. https://www.pregnancymagazine.com/pregnancy/emergency-birth-cant-get-to-hospital

Marcin, A. (2019, October 2). *What Is Hypnobirthing? Technique, How-To, Pros and Cons.* Healthline. https://www.healthline.com/health/pregnancy/hypnobirthing

Masters, M. (2021, June 22). *Can You Take Baths While Pregnant?* What to Expect. https://www.whattoexpect.com/pregnancy/looking-good/pampered-parts/bathing.aspx#bath

Masters, M. (2022, February 22). *Is Your Hair Falling Out?* What to Expect. https://www.whattoexpect.com/first-year/postpartum-health-and-care/postpartum-hair-loss/

Matta, C. (2022, October 30). *Can I Get Botox While Pregnant?* Verywell Family. https://www.verywellfamily.com/can-i-get-botox-when-pregnant-5198014#:~:text=Risks%20of%20Using%20Botox%20While%20Pregnant

May I break your waters? Information on Artificial Rupture of Membranes. (2014, June 12). Aimsireland. http://aimsireland.ie/may-i-break-your-waters-information-on-artificial-rupture-of-membranes-2/

McTigue, S. (2020, March 26). *What Are the Earliest Signs of Being Pregnant with Twins?* Healthline. https://www.healthline.com/health/pregnancy/signs-of-twins#chances-of-twins

Medications for Pain Relief During Labor and Delivery. (2022, December 4). ACOG. https://www.acog.org/womens-health/faqs/medications-for-pain-relief-during-labor-and-delivery#:~:text=An%20epidural%20block%20(also%20called

Medicines During Pregnancy. (2022, February 23). Myhealth https://myhealth.alberta.ca/Health/Pages/conditions.aspx?hwid=uf9707#:~:text=Deciding%20about%20medicines%20during%20pregnancy

Miles, K. (2021, February 4). *Forceps delivery and vacuum delivery.* BabyCenter. https://www.babycenter.com/pregnancy/your-body/forceps-and-vacuum-deliveries_1451360

Moderate Amounts of Caffeine Not Linked to Maternal Health Risks. (2021, November 11). Pennmedicine.org. https://www.pennmedicine.org/news/news-releases/2021/november/moderate-amounts-of-caffeine-not-linked-to-maternal-health-risks

Moldenhauer, J. S. (2022, September 3). *Prelabor Rupture of the Membranes (PROM).* Women's Health Issues: MSD Manual Consumer Version https://www.msdmanuals.com/home/women-s-health-issues/complications-of-labor-and-delivery/prelabor-rupture-of-the-membranes-prom

Movement and positions during labour. (n.d.). Tommys https://www.tommys.org/pregnancy-information/giving-birth/movement-and-positions-during-labour

Myths: Smoking and Pregnancy | Smokefree Women. (2019, June 1). Smokefree.gov. https://women.smokefree.gov/pregnancy-motherhood/quitting-while-pregnant/myths-about-smoking-pregnancy

Nair, A. (2020, October 27). *Postnatal Examination: Purpose, Check Ups, Questions to Ask.* Parenting.firstcry.com. https://parenting.firstcry.com/articles/your-postnatal-examination-what-to-expect/

Nall, R. (2016, November 28). *Placenta Delivery: What to Expect.* Healthline Media. https://www.healthline.com/health/pregnancy/placenta-delivery

Navsaria, D. (2020, March 3). *Bathing Your Baby.* HealthyChildren.org. https://www.healthychildren.org/English/ages-stages/baby/bathing-skin-care/Pages/Bathing-Your-Newborn.aspx#:~:text=The%20World%20Health%20Organization%20(WHO

Newborn screening tests for your baby. (2020, July). March of Dimes. https://www.marchofdimes.org/find-support/topics/parenthood/newborn-screening-tests-your-baby

Nguyen, H. (2021, September 29). *Postpartum recovery: What to expect.* HealthPartners Blog.

https://www.healthpartners.com/blog/what-to-expect-after-giving-birth/

Ogunyemi, D. (2022, January). *Bonding With Your Newborn: What to Know If You Don't Feel Connected Right Away.* Acog.org. https://www.acog.org/womens-health/experts-and-stories/the-latest/bonding-with-your-newborn-heres-what-to-know-if-you-dont-feel-connected-right-away#:~:text=Many%20new%0Oparents%20need%20m ore

Opt-Out| Pregnant Women, Infants, and Children. (2019). Centers for Disease Control and Prevention. https://www.cdc.gov/hiv/group/gender/pregnantwo men/opt-out.html

Overview - Newborn jaundice. (2019). NHS. https://www.nhs.uk/conditions/Jaundice-newborn/

Pacheko, D. (2020, October 30). *Pregnancy & Sleep: Tips, Sleep Positions, & Issues.* Sleep Foundation. https://www.sleepfoundation.org/pregnancy#:~:text= Common%20Sleep%20Disorders%20and%20Problem s%20During%20Pregnancy.%20The

Pain relief in labour. (2020, December 2). NHS https://www.nhs.uk/pregnancy/labour-and-birth/what-happens/pain-relief-in-labour/

Patient Information Induction of Labour. (2017). NHS https://www.hdft.nhs.uk/content/uploads/2018/07/B irth-Induction-of-Labour-leaflet.pdf

Pearl, E., & Joseph, B. (2022, March 5). *Can I Still Drink Coffee While I'm Pregnant? (for Parents).* Nemours KidsHealth. https://kidshealth.org/en/parents/preg-caffeine.html

Perineal massage during pregnancy. (2021, November 22). HSE.ie. https://www2.hse.ie/pregnancy-birth/labour/preparing/perineal-massage-during-pregnancy/

Placenta praevia (low-lying placenta). (2021, February 26). HSE.ie. https://www2.hse.ie/conditions/placenta-praevia/#:~:text=Placenta%20praevia%20happens%20when%20the

Placental abruption - Symptoms and causes. (2022, February 25). Mayo Clinic. https://www.mayoclinic.org/diseases-conditions/placental-abruption/symptoms-causes/syc-20376458#:~:text=Placental%20abruption%20occurs%20when%20the%20placenta%20partly%20or%20completely%20separates

Pollack, S. (2021, September 9). *HR Headaches: When and How Should I Tell My Employer That I'm Pregnant?* Workest. https://www.zenefits.com/workest/hr-headaches-when-and-how-should-i-tell-my-employer-that-im-pregnant/#:~:text=baby

Postpartum Depression - Symptoms and Causes. (2018b, September 1). Mayo Clinic. https://www.mayoclinic.org/diseases-conditions/postpartum-depression/symptoms-causes/syc-20376617

Postpartum Emotional Deluge. (n.d.). Bodily. https://itsbodily.com/blogs/birth-recovery-postpartum/postpartum-emotions-changes-after-giving-birth

Postpartum Preeclampsia: Risk after Delivery Remains. (2019, May 29). DONA International. https://www.dona.org/postpartum-preeclampsia-risk-after-delivery-remains/#:~:text=Unfortunately%2C%2075%25%20of%20maternal%20deaths

Pregnancy 101. (2019). National Geographic [Video]. YouTube. https://www.youtube.com/watch?v=XEfnq4Q4bfk+B 5:B29

Pregnancy and Bladder Control. (2020, November 6). Cleveland Clinic. https://my.clevelandclinic.org/health/articles/16094-pregnancy-and-bladder-control

Pregnancy and Heartburn. (2015, May 3). Cleveland Clinic. https://my.clevelandclinic.org/health/diseases/12011-heartburn-during-pregnancy

Pregnancy Emotions & Mood Swings: Challenges Every New Parent Faces. (2018, June 16). ForWhen. https://forwhenhelpline.org.au/parent-resources/pregnancy-emotions-mood-swings/#:~:text=The%20third%20trimester%20can%20be

Pregnancy Glossary: Your A to Z Guide to Pregnancy Terminology. (n.d.). What to Expect. https://www.whattoexpect.com/pregnancy/glossary

Pregnancy nutrition: Foods to avoid. (2017, March 31). Mayo Clinic. https://www.mayoclinic.org/healthy-lifestyle/pregnancy-week-by-week/in-depth/pregnancy-nutrition/art-20043844

Pregnancy Stretch Marks: Prevention & Treatment. (2022, July 11). Web-Pampers-US-EN. https://www.pampers.com/en-us/pregnancy/pregnancy-symptoms/article/pregnancy-stretch-marks

Pregnancy Weight Gain Calculator. (2009, March 8). Calculator.net. https://www.calculator.net/pregnancy-weight-gain-calculator.html

Pregnancy. (2021, May 4). ADA. https://www.ada.org/resources/research/science-and-research-institute/oral-health-topics/pregnancy

Prenatal care checkups. (2017, June 18). March of Dimes. https://www.marchofdimes.org/find-support/topics/planning-baby/prenatal-care-checkups

Prenatal care: 1st trimester visits. (2018, August 6). Mayo Clinic. https://www.mayoclinic.org/healthy-lifestyle/pregnancy-week-by-week/in-depth/prenatal-care/art-20044882

Prenatal care: 2nd trimester visits. (2022, August 4). Mayo Clinic. https://www.mayoclinic.org/healthy-lifestyle/pregnancy-week-by-week/in-depth/prenatal-care/art-20044581

Prenatal Care—The Full Guide. (n.d.). Pampers https://www.pampers.com/en-us/pregnancy/prenatal-health-and-wellness/article/prenatal-care

Prenatal screening for genetic conditions. (n.d.). Department of Health Australia. https://www.healthywa.wa.gov.au/Articles/N_R/Pren atal-screening-for-genetic-conditions

Prenatal testing: Is it right for you? (2020, August 25). Mayo Clinic. https://www.mayoclinic.org/healthy-lifestyle/pregnancy-week-by-week/in-depth/prenatal-testing/art-20045177

Preparing baby formula. (2022, November 10). HSE.ie. https://www2.hse.ie/babies-children/bottle-feeding/preparing-baby-formula/

PUPPP Rash: Symptoms, Causes, Treatment & Prevention. (2022, February 9). Cleveland Clinic. https://my.clevelandclinic.org/health/diseases/22374-puppp-rash#:~:text=PUPPP%20is%20an%20itchy%20rash

Recovering after an episiotomy. (2019, June 19). HSE.ie. https://www2.hse.ie/pregnancy-birth/birth/episiotomy/recovering/

Recovering from a perineal tear. (n.d.-c). Tommys. https://www.tommys.org/pregnancy-information/after-birth/recovering-perineal-tear

Rh Factor Blood Type and Pregnancy. (2020, April 27). American Pregnancy Association. https://americanpregnancy.org/healthy-pregnancy/pregnancy-complications/rh-factor

Richardson, J. H., & Littleton, K. (2015). *Breastfeeding FAQs: How Much and How Often (for Parents).* KidsHealth.

https://kidshealth.org/en/parents/breastfeed-often.html

Ridgeon, E. (2021, May 7). *Spinal anaesthesia in labour and childbirth.* My BabyManual. https://mybabymanual.co.uk/childbirth/delivery/spinal-anaesthesia-in-labour-and-childbirth/

Rigsby, K. (2019, December 13). *I'm Pregnant. When Should I Go to the Doctor?* Ntmconline.net. https://ntmconline.net/im-pregnant-when-should-i-go-to-the-doctor/

Riley, L. (2009, November 3). *Q&A: What Happens If I Can't Make it to the Hospital?* Parents. https://www.parents.com/pregnancy/my-life/emotions/qa-what-happens-if-i-cant-make-it-to-the-hospital/

Romito, K., Bailey, T. M., Husney, A., & Jones, K. (2022, February 23). *Breathing Techniques for Childbirth.* Myhealth.alberta.ca. https://myhealth.alberta.ca/Health/pages/conditions.aspx?hwid=tn7421

Rosenblum, N. (n.d.). *Breastfeeding 101: Q&A with Lactation Expert Nadine Rosenblum.* Hopkinsmedicine.org. https://www.hopkinsmedicine.org/health/wellness-and-prevention/breastfeeding-101-qanda-with-lactation-expert-nadine-rosenblum

Ruddy, E. Z. (2022, May 6). *9 Surprising Truths About Postpartum Sex After Birth.* Parents. https://www.parents.com/parenting/relationships/sex

-and-marriage-after-baby/how-to-have-great-postpartum-sex/

Savchenko, M. (2019, July 9). *How to Prepare for Breastfeeding Before Your Baby Arrives.* Flo.health - #1 Mobile Product for Women's Health. https://flo.health/being-a-mom/your-baby/baby-care-and-feeding/how-to-prepare-for-breastfeeding#:~:text=Most%20obstetricians%20and%20lactation%20consultants

Sex after pregnancy: Set your own timeline. (2022, December 6). Mayo Clinic. https://www.mayoclinic.org/healthy-lifestyle/labor-and-delivery/in-depth/sex-after-pregnancy/art-20045669#:~:text=While%20there

Sex in trimester one, two and three of pregnancy | Pregnancy articles & support. (2022, August 18). National Childbirth Trust. https://www.nct.org.uk/pregnancy/relationships-sex/sex-trimester-one-two-and-three-pregnancy

Sickle Cell Disease. (n.d.). Johns Hopkins Medicine https://www.hopkinsmedicine.org/health/conditions-and-diseases/sickle-cell-disease#:~:text=Sickle%20cell%20disease%20is%20an%20inherited%20blood%20disorder%20marked%20by

Silver, E. (2019, January 16). *Why you shouldn't shave down there before labour.* Today's Parent. https://www.todaysparent.com/pregnancy/giving-birth/why-you-shouldnt-shave-down-there-before-labour/

Slaughter, E. (2019). *What are the Effects & Dangers of Alcohol During Pregnancy?* American Addiction Centers.

https://americanaddictioncenters.org/alcoholism-treatment/dangers-pregnancy

Smyth, R., Markham, C., & Dowswell, T. (2013, June 18). *Amniotomy for shortening spontaneous labour.* Cochrane.org. https://www.cochrane.org/CD006167/PREG_amniotomy-for-shortening-spontaneous-labour

Stages of labour. (2023, January 4). HSE.ie. https://www2.hse.ie/pregnancy-birth/labour/preparing/stages-labour

Stein, E., Gordon, S., & Riley, L. (2022, December 19). *Signs of Approaching Labor: How to Tell Your Baby is Coming Soon.* Parents. https://www.parents.com/pregnancy/giving-birth/signs-of-labor/signs-of-approaching-labor/

Sumner, C. (2005, October 3). *8 Marriage Issues You'll Face After Baby and How to Solve Them.* Parents. https://www.parents.com/parenting/relationships/staying-close/marriage-after-baby/

Swollen ankles, feet and fingers in pregnancy. (2019, May 17). HSE.ie. https://www2.hse.ie/conditions/swollen-ankles-feet-fingers-pregnancy/

Ten tips for birth partners. (2020, December 2). National Childbirth Trust. https://www.nct.org.uk/labour-birth/dads-and-partners/ten-tips-for-birth-partners

Terreri, C. (2013, October 20). *How to Use Water for Comfort in Labor.* Lamaze International. https://www.lamaze.org/Giving-Birth-with-Confidence/GBWC-Post/how-to-use-water-for-comfort-in-labor

The Essential Hospital Bag Checklist. (2022, November). My
    Expert   Midwife.
    https://myexpertmidwife.ie/blogs/my-expert-
    midwife/essential-items-for-your-hosp

Think You Can't Breastfeed After Implants? Think Again. (2021a,
    August   8).   Johns   Hopkins   Medicine.
    https://www.hopkinsmedicine.org/health/wellness-
    and-prevention/think-you-cant-breastfeed-after-
    implants-think-again

Thomas, L. (2017, August 8). *Labor: what is the "show"?* News-
    Medical.net.   https://www.news-
    medical.net/health/Labor-what-is-the-show.aspx

Timing your contractions - when to go to the hospital. (2023, January 4).
    HSE.ie.   https://www2.hse.ie/pregnancy-
    birth/labour/signs-labour/timing-your-contractions/

Today's Parent. (2018). *What to expect in your First Trimester of
    pregnancy | Pregnancy Week-by-Week* [Video]. YouTube.
    https://www.youtube.com/watch?v=cfn04QUO4B8

Todd, N. (2017, February 13). *How Can I Handle My Labor Pain?*
    WebMD.
    https://www.webmd.com/baby/guide/pregnancy-
    pain-relief

Toxoplasma from Food Safety for Moms to Be. (2020). FDA.
    https://www.fda.gov/food/people-risk-foodborne-
    illness/toxoplasma-food-safety-moms-be

Traveling While Pregnant or Breastfeeding. (2020, February 11).
    Johns   Hopkins   Medicine.

https://www.hopkinsmedicine.org/health/conditions-and-diseases/traveling-while-pregnant-or-breastfeeding

Umbilical cord care: Do's and don'ts for parents. (2022, February 24). Mayo Clinic. https://www.mayoclinic.org/healthy-lifestyle/infant-and-toddler-health/in-depth/umbilical-cord/art-20048250#:~:text=A%20baby

Understand how COVID-19 might affect your pregnancy. (2022, September 7). Mayo Clinic. https://www.mayoclinic.org/diseases-conditions/coronavirus/in-depth/pregnancy-and-covid-19/art-20482639

Understand the symptoms of depression during pregnancy. (2019, June 5). Mayo Clinic. https://www.mayoclinic.org/healthy-lifestyle/pregnancy-week-by-week/in-depth/depression-during-pregnancy/art-20237875

University of Michigan (2020). A randomized controlled trial of the hypnoBirthing program: Effects on labor, stress and pain. *BMC Pregnancy and Childbirth, 20*(1), 1-10. doi:10.1186/s12884-020-27040-6

Vaccination Considerations for People who are Pregnant or Breastfeeding. (2020, February 11). Centers for Disease Control and Prevention. https://www.cdc.gov/coronavirus/2019-ncov/vaccines/recommendations/pregnancy.html

Vaginal Birth After Cesarean (VBAC): Facts, Safety & Risks. (2021, August 23). Cleveland Clinic. https://my.clevelandclinic.org/health/articles/21687-vaginal-birth-after-cesarean-vbac#:~:text=If%20you

Varicose Veins During Pregnancy: Types, Causes & Treatment. (2022c, May 25). Cleveland Clinic. https://my.clevelandclinic.org/health/diseases/23331-varicose-veins-in-pregnancy

Vitamins and supplements during pregnancy. (2022b, October 17). Healthdirect Australia. https://www.pregnancybirthbaby.org.au/vitamins-and-supplements-during-pregnancy#vitamins-and-minerals

Water Births (2017, April 26). American Pregnancy Association. https://americanpregnancy.org/healthy-pregnancy/labor-and-birth/water-births/#:~:text=Benefits%20for%20Mother%3A&text=Buoyancy%20promotes%20more%20efficient%20uterine,blood%20pressure%20caused%20by%20anxiety.

Watson, S. (2021, December 2). *Coping with pregnancy loss.* BabyCenter. https://www.babycenter.com/pregnancy/your-life/coping-with-pregnancy-loss_4006

Weiss, R. E. (2021, September 13). *How to Combat Boredom During a Long Labor.* Verywell Family. https://www.verywellfamily.com/things-to-do-during-labor-to-prevent-boredom-4111058

When breastfeeding or feeding expressed milk is not recommended. (2019c, December 14). Centers for Disease Control and Prevention. https://www.cdc.gov/breastfeeding/breastfeeding-special-circumstances/contraindications-to-breastfeeding.html

When Is It Safe to Deliver Your Baby? (2020). University of Utah. https://healthcare.utah.edu/womenshealth/pregnancy-birth/preterm-birth/when-is-it-safe-to-deliver.php

Wild, S., & Nierenberg, C. (2018, March 27). *Vaginal Birth vs. C-Section: Pros & Cons.* Live Science. https://www.livescience.com/45681-vaginal-birth-vs-c-section.html

Your antenatal appointment schedule. (n.d.). Tommy's. https://www.tommys.org/pregnancy-information/im-pregnant/antenatal-care/your-antenatal-appointment-schedule

Your body after the birth (the first 6 weeks). (n.d.). Tommy's. https://www.tommys.org/pregnancy-information/after-birth/your-body-after-birth

Your postpartum checkups. (2018, July). March of Dimes. https://www.marchofdimes.org/find-support/topics/postpartum/your-postpartum-checkup

Image References

Mendes, L. (2021). *Breastfeeding baby* [Image]. Unsplash. **https://unsplash.com/photos/L0cDMFldZgg**

Notes

Notes

Notes

Notes

Notes

Notes

Notes

Notes

Notes

Notes

Notes

Notes

Milton Keynes UK
Ingram Content Group UK Ltd.
UKHW020953221123
433051UK00021B/1255